THE NATURAL FACELIFT

THE NATURAL FACELIFT

JOSEPH CORVO

CENTURY

LONDON SYDNEY AUCKLAND JOHANNESBURG

Published in 1991 by Century
Random Century Ltd
20 Vauxhall Bridge Road, London SW1V 2SA

Random Century Australia (Pty) Ltd
20 Alfred Street, Milsons Point, Sydney, NSW 2061, Australia

Random Century New Zealand Ltd
9–11 Rothwell Avenue, Albany, Auckland 10, New Zealand

Random Century South Africa (Pty) Ltd
PO Box 337, Bergvlei 2012, South Africa

Joseph Corvo's right to be identified as the author of this work has been
asserted by him in accordance with the Copyright, Designs and Patents
Act, 1988.

Set in 11/13 Century Lasercomp
Printed and bound in U.K. by
Butler & Tanner Ltd, Frome and London

A catalogue record for this book is available from the British Library.

ISBN 0–7126–4756–2

CONTENTS

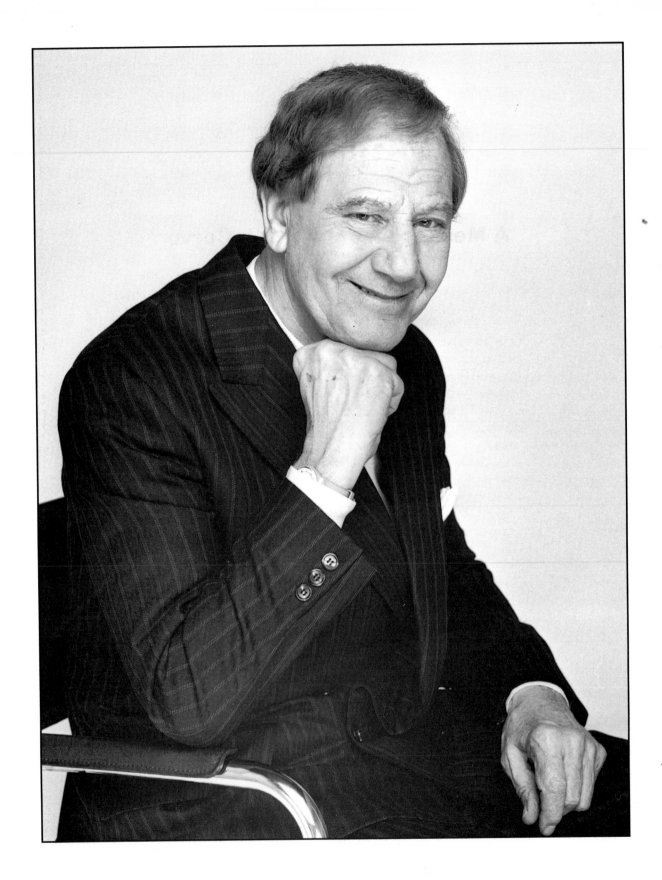

A Message from Joseph Corvo

From this moment your life is going to change. Ageing has always been looked on as inevitable, but there is a way out: Zone Therapy.

If you spend just ten minutes a day practising my face plan, you can have all the benefits of Zone Therapy: the youth, health and beauty that comes from glands and organs working to 100 per cent efficiency.

If you are willing to spend an extra ten minutes practising my NATURAL FACELIFT, you can mould the contours of your face to the shape you desire, cleanse your skin from the inside and on the outside to be clear, smooth and glowing with health, and make the miraculous youth that Zone Therapy gives you shine through your eyes.

And if you are willing to follow the Zone Therapy lifestyle through the rest of the day you can stay young into your eighties, prevent illness and enjoy the sex secrets of Zone Therapy. I will give you a lifetime's sense of total fulfilment and deep happiness.

Surgery can give you a beauty that is only skin deep. It can only alter the contours of your face. How often do we see women who have had surgical facelifts whose faces are just dead slabs of skin or stretched, lifeless masks from behind which stare frightened, elderly eyes. Zone Therapy not only moulds the contours of the face, but gives you the true animating beauty that comes from deep within, shining out of sparkling eyes and glorious skin.

You needn't lose your looks. You needn't lose your dignity trying to keep them. Be your age, but be the best for your age.

Joseph Corvo

1

ZONE THERAPY AGAINST AGEING

The Zone Therapy revolution is beginning. For over thirty years now I have been treating private patients, including some of the world's most beautiful women (and some of its most handsome men). I have shown them how to stay young, beautiful and healthy into their eighties by practising Zone Therapy's simple system of pressure point massage for just ten minutes a day.

Last year I decided that the secrets of Zone Therapy ought to be available to everyone, not just the rich and famous, so I published my first book, *Joseph Corvo's Zone Therapy*. It became an immediate international bestseller. One of the aspects of this success which has most pleased me is the way the popularity of Zone Therapy is spreading by word of mouth.

This is because Zone Therapy works.

How does it work? Well, Zone Therapy is the science of bringing to perfection the body's natural powers of regeneration. In this sense Zone Therapy's method of healing is as old as mankind. If you hurt yourself, your first instinct is always to rub the painful part with your hand. Pressure gives comfort. Moreover through the centuries certain healers have worked miracles by the laying on of hands. But never before has the scientific basis for these phenomena been worked out, or the most effective application of these natural powers been put into a system. That system is Zone Therapy.

Because we eat impure foods, breathe impure air, and particularly if we eat or smoke or drink excessively, impurities enter the systems. Nerve endings silt up with the result that the electro-magnetic forces which nourish and regenerate the body's vital glands and organs become sluggish. Each year we lose a little more power. When we are twenty-five years old our glands and organs are normally 100 per cent efficient, but from then on, starved of the natural power of renewal by increasing blockage of the systems, they cut back steadily to 90 per cent, 80 per cent

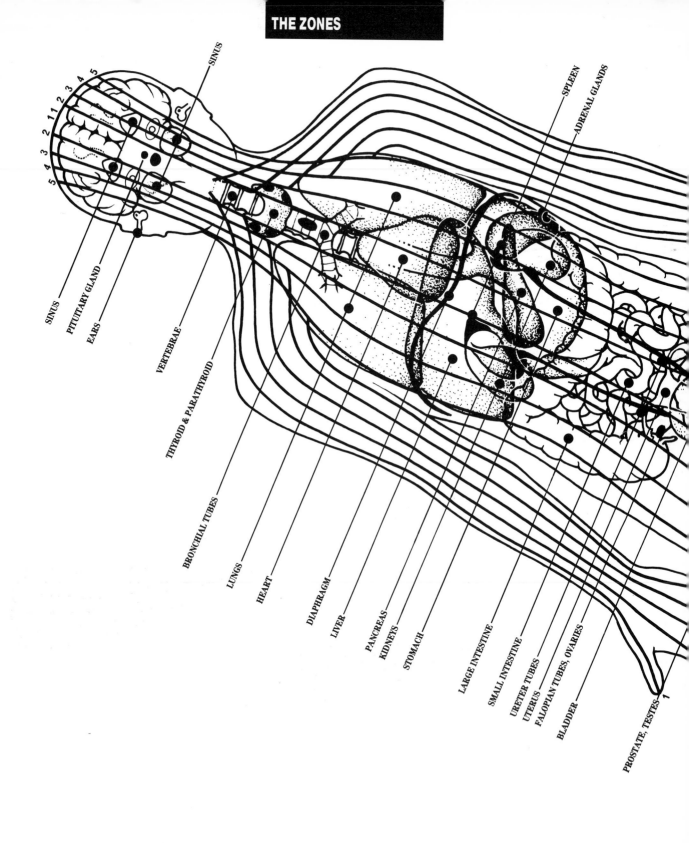

10

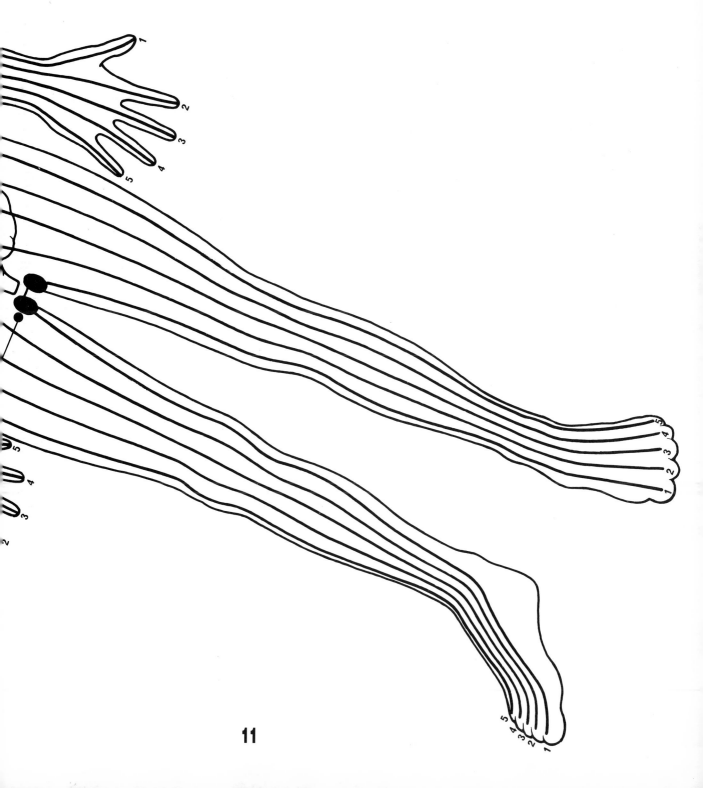

and so on. Illnesses arise as glands and organs malfunction. Eventually 30 per cent efficiency brings senility and death.

Zone Therapy is a system of pressure point massage which works by dispersing the toxins that have accumulated on the terminal nerve endings, particularly on the hands, feet and face, so that the glands and organs are brought up to 100 per cent efficiency again. The regenerating electro-magnetic forces power round the ten zones of your body, renewing the glands and organs in their respective zones. You become as healthy,

Pressure points – the hands

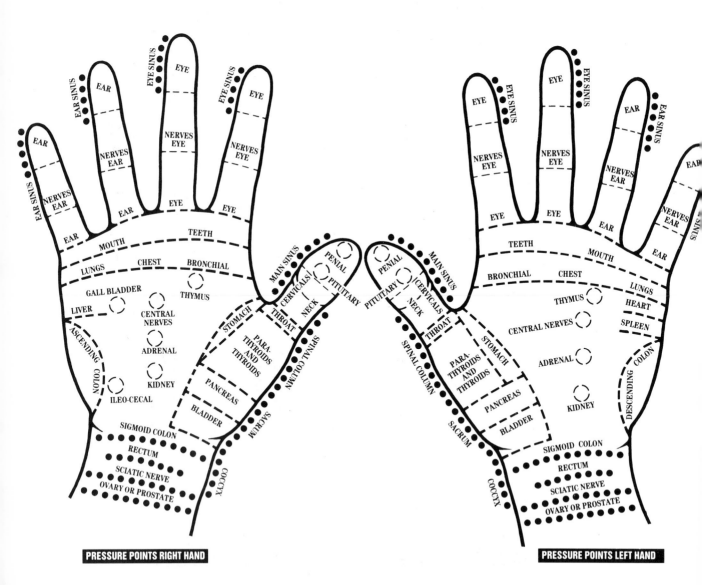

PRESSURE POINTS RIGHT HAND

PRESSURE POINTS LEFT HAND

youthful and beautiful as it is possible for you to be. A sixty year old can feel as young and healthy as a forty year old, a forty year old can look like a thirty year old.

Zone Therapy has two main uses. First, the basic ten minutes a day tone up, if rigorously kept to, can bring about an amazing improvement in your general state of health and feeling of well-being. Only Zone Therapy can give you the true health that comes from within; while

Pressure points – the feet

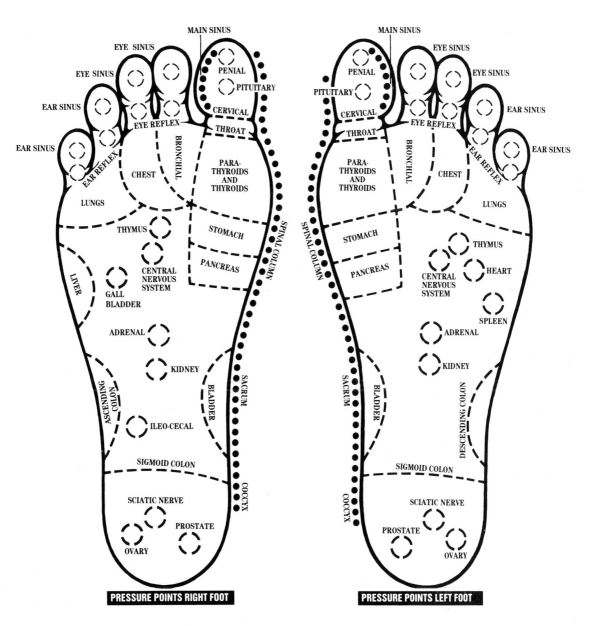

millions of people spend hours every week jogging or working out, the results they achieve will only be superficial so long as they fail to exercise as well their inner selves, i.e. their organs and their glands. Only Zone Therapy can reach these. Second, Zone Therapy can be aimed in a definite and distinct direction such as towards healing a particular illness or keeping or regaining youth – and it is to this particular end that many of my most famous clients come to see me. With Zone Therapy you can simply press away the years.

Ageing is in fact a form of illness, because it is due entirely to wearing down of the glandular and organic systems.

If you are twenty-five or younger and you practise Zone Therapy, you need never age.

If you do not practise Zone Therapy from the age of twenty-five onwards, then the decline in your glandular and organic systems will begin to cause a drying of the facial skin, usually at the sides of the eyes. Muscle wastage will occur as your muscles fail to receive 100 per cent regenerative power. Deterioration of facial muscle then leads to hollow cheeks around the cheek bones and a flabbiness around the cheeks, which droop around the mouth. Lines appear around the corners of the mouth and jowls loosen. After forty, loose skin makes you look pounds heavier even if you are not. Muscle wastage causes a droop and a definite thickening of the stomach area. Wrinkles show even through half a ton of make-up. You develop a turkey neck, and your eyelids and the skin above your eyes hangs loose.

In addition to the toxins eaten or breathed in, the process of premature ageing is usually accelerated even further by stress, depression and boredom. Stress has the effect of emptying the adrenal glands so that you become tired and depressed, and a malfunction will then spread through the more closely related glands – the endocrine, the liver, the spleen, the kidneys and the thymus. Complete disintegration of the body and spirit results.

If some glands and organs deteriorate more quickly than others because, for example, of particular abuses such as smoking, excess drinking or bad eating habits, then special problems will arise in the process of ageing, such as spots, broken veins, facial hair, flaky skin, excess fat, bags under the eyes, cloudy eyes, etc.

If, on the other hand, you practise Zone Therapy on a daily basis your face remains firm and even. Your skin is clean, smooth, moist and tight. Your muscles remain flexible, elastic and precise in contour. Your eyes are bright and full of life. Work at the exercises as instructed in this book and you will be truly amazed at the results. Of course, you can't stop the ageing process, but you can certainly slow it down almost to a standstill. Work at it every day and you can look ten or even twenty years younger. If you are twenty years old now and you start to look after yourself, then at the age of fifty you can still look thirty.

Some people will tell you that you can rejuvenate your skin by what

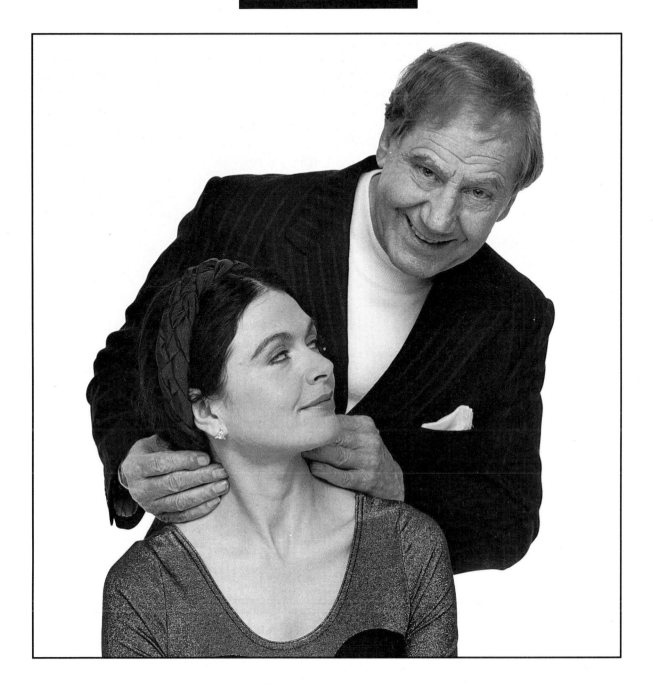

you apply to it. Unfortunately nothing that you put on your face can nourish it. There are no magic cures for ageing *apart from the body's own miraculous powers*. Neither can true beauty come from the knife. It comes from within in two senses. Firstly, because it depends on glandular and organic perfection, and secondly, because it depends on the attractive, glad-to-be-alive feeling which comes from that perfection.

So I repeat: there is a way out: Zone Therapy. Be determined, be positive, and Zone Therapy will save you.

15

CHAPTER 2

JOSEPH CORVO'S NATURAL FACELIFT

LOSE TEN YEARS IN TWENTY MINUTES A DAY

What I'm about to show you will have a dramatic effect on your face. It will cleanse the skin on the inside and the outside, exercise your outer self, your muscles, your glands and organs. It will give you inner and outer radiance and instil in you the deepest relaxation you have ever known.

I must emphasize that Zone Therapy is the key to everything that follows; the muscle-building exercises, the relaxation techniques, the skin-care advice and the dietary recommendations will only be 20 per cent effective if they are not practised with a daily 15 pressure point massage of ten minutes.

So, I am going to tell you how to cleanse your skin on the outside so that your pores remain clear and the texture of your skin neither flaky nor greasy. I am going to tell you how to cleanse your skin on the inside, purifying the blood so that your skin remains clear and without spots or blemishes. Stress accelerates the ageing process beyond belief, so I am going to teach you to relax, so that rather than wasting your body's natural energies on fruitless worrying, you can direct them towards rejuvenating yourself. Most visible ageing is caused by muscle wastage, which occurs when terminal nerve endings become blocked with the result that the regenerative electro-magnetic forces do not carry the necessary energy to the muscles. I am going to show you how to reopen the channels so that the muscles receive all the nourishment they need, and then show you how to build your facial muscles so that they are as firm and finely shaped as you would wish. I am going to show you how to empty the lymph glands in your face, where excess liquid is stored, and how to work directly on the veins and arteries that carry nourishing blood and oxygen and remove unhealthy waste matter from the skin. I am going to show you how to work directly on the skin in order to tone it up, how to invigorate it and remove the uppermost layer of dead skin. Finally, I am going to tell you the correct creams to use to make your skin as young as a twenty-five year old's.

You are going to see dramatic results.

Practise every day. Make sure you have the time without feeling rushed.

CLEANSING

Bare your face, neck and shoulders then thoroughly cleanse your skin.

The skin is self-cleansing and self-nourishing by a process that comes from the inside, so the washing you do on a daily basis is to remove dirt, grime and excess sebum. Never be rough on your face with a towel or rub it abrasively.

If you have to wash with a soap then use a mild unperfumed one. Before you put soap on your face make sure your hands are clean otherwise the dirt from your hands ends up on your face. If you have a dry skin you need a soap high in fat content.

Rinse your face very well, then splash with cold water, then pat your face dry with a towel. Do not rub it dry.

Most foundations for the face like powders, blushers and make-up are water soluble and can easily be removed with soap and water. If you find that particles of make-up are still clinging to your face, you should use a cleanser. Some types of make-up for face and eyes require a cream or liquid cleanser. If your skin is oily, choose a light cleansing milk. If your skin tends to be dry, choose a richer cleansing cream.

Start your cleansing ritual from your neck upwards, using as much cotton wool as you need to do a good job. Use firm upward strokes and follow up with a good toner.

Make gentle sweeping strokes to remove dirt and grease.

RELAXING

Stress wastes the body's natural regenerating power and distracts the mind from the concentration of will needed for total effectiveness in the practice of Zone Therapy. Stress causes the heart to beat faster so that blood pressure increases, the digestive system is disturbed and the nervous system is strained. The result is that there is a tremendous amount of wear and tear on our muscles and internal organs. If we are stressed, we spend more energy keeping the muscles in continual readiness for work than we do actually working. Stress is terribly ageing – it always shows directly on the face.

The following exercises, which you need to perform for a total of five minutes (one minute per exercise), will not only give you a lovely feeling of half floating out of your body, but in the pressure point massage and face-building exercises that follow, they will enable you to concentrate on the pressure point or lymph gland or muscle specified so that you can achieve the most amazing results.

Arm Stretch

Stand up erect, feet about 12 inches apart, arms outstretched at shoulder level. Gently close your hand into a fist, loosely not tight.

Rotate shoulders, back and down, away from your ears. Keep your arms at shoulder level, don't let them drop. As you will feel, this exercise takes the strain off the lower back and releases tension in the neck. Look straight ahead, do not drop your head. Perform for one minute.

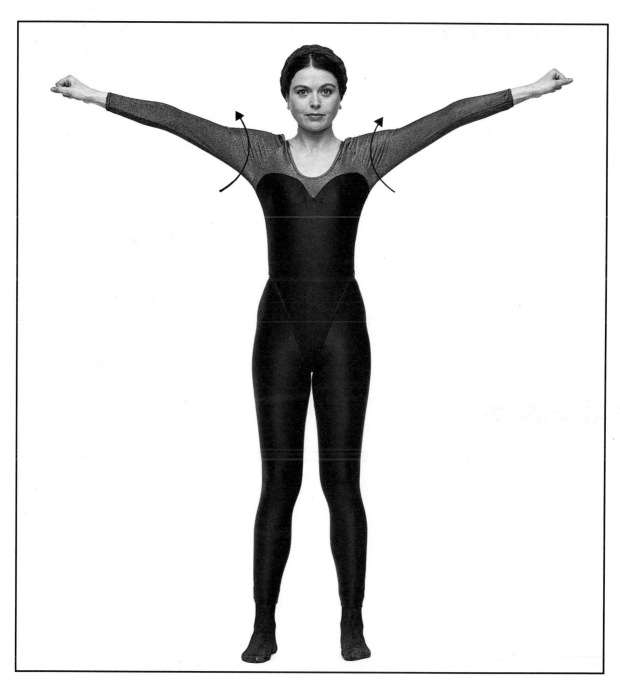

The Tree Exercise

Stand up against the wall for this exercise until you have mastered it. Once you are well balanced you can do it anywhere.

Look at the photo carefully. Then, standing absolutely straight, leave one foot on the floor and the other foot resting as far up as you can on the inner thighs. Arms stretched up above you reaching as far as you can. Hold for ten seconds and then change, so if your right foot is on the ground to start with, your left foot will be on your right thigh, so you change to left foot on the ground, right foot on left thigh every ten seconds. Change over for period of one minute.

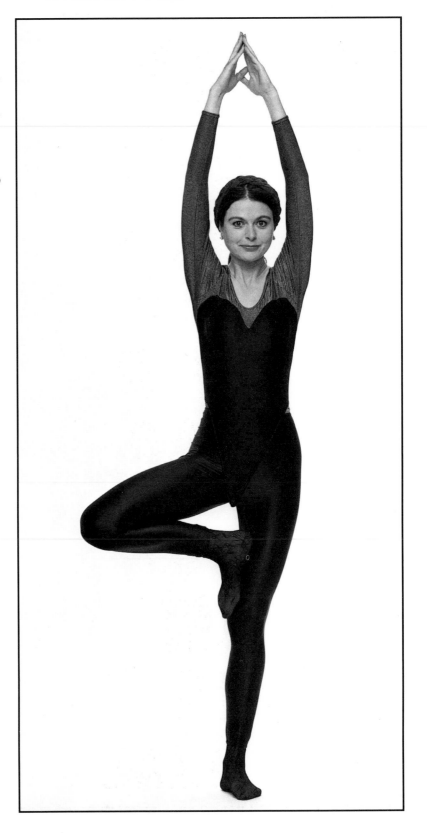

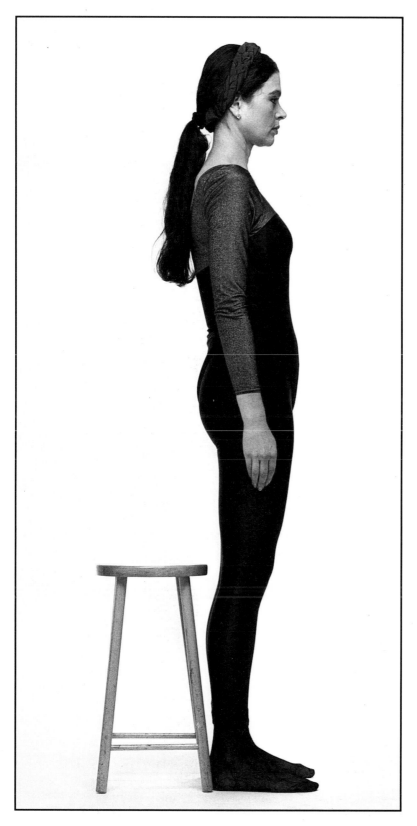

Neck Stretch
To sit down properly takes practice. So stand with your back to the stool.

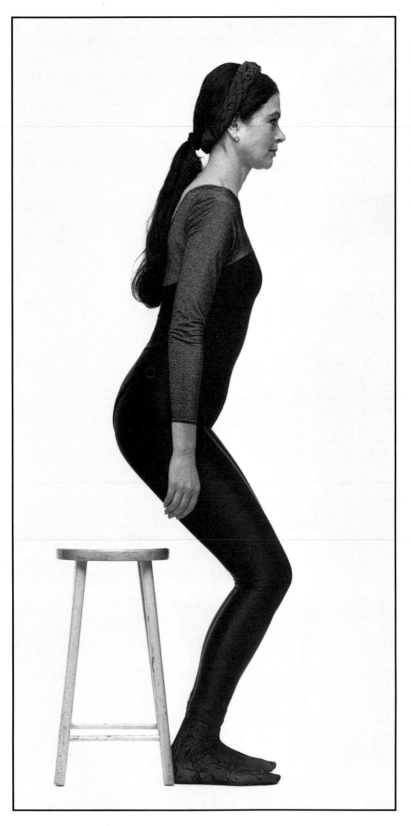

Bend your knees and place your buttocks on the stool as described in the photograph. Feet must be 12 inches apart, both feet on the ground, your back perfectly straight, head held level, arms hanging loosely by your sides. This exercise is to give maximum relaxation to the head, neck and shoulders.

Put your buttocks well back on the stool, your weight evenly distributed on both buttocks. Do not cross your ankles or your knees because you cut down the blood circulation to and from your legs and throw terrific strain on your spine; your bodyline is also badly affected. Keep the thighs parallel.

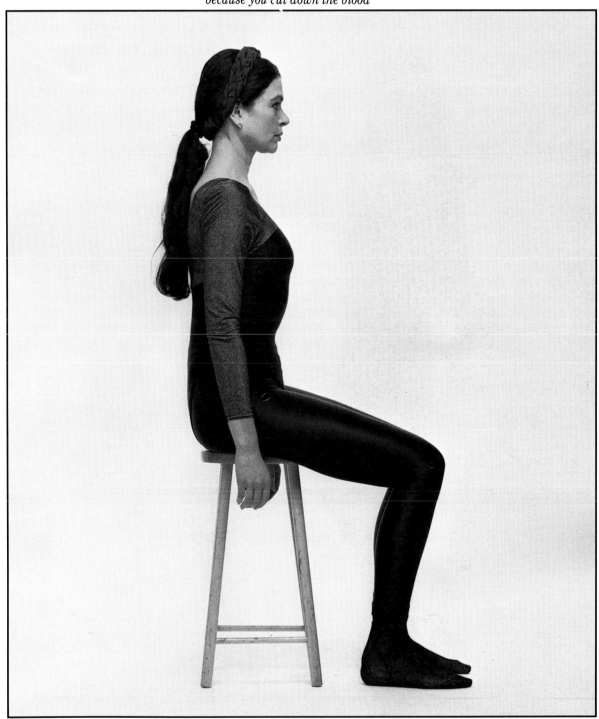

Your neck supports the weight of your head and acts as a pathway for the central nervous system, blood circulation and vessels, your respiratory and digestive systems.

It transmits messages from the brain to parts of the body. Tension produced by stress often results in the head being held incorrectly either too far forward or too far

back and too much on one side, so further tension is created in the muscles that connect the head to the shoulders. These exercises are designed to rectify that condition.

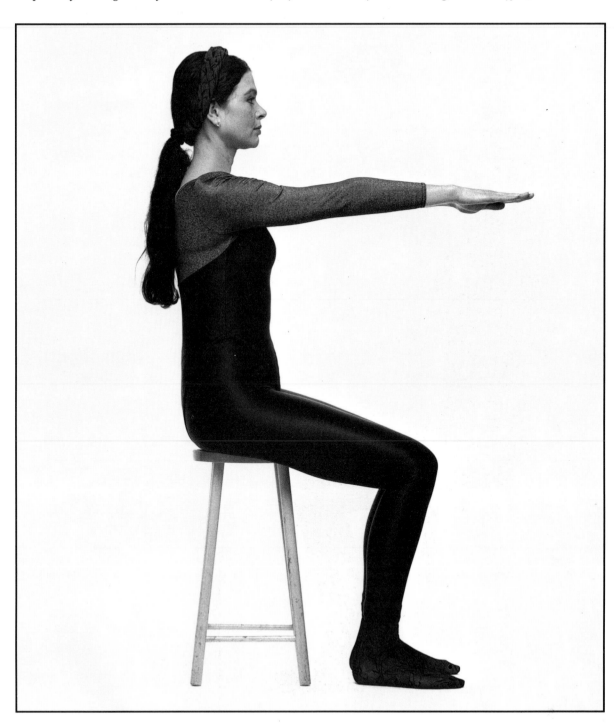

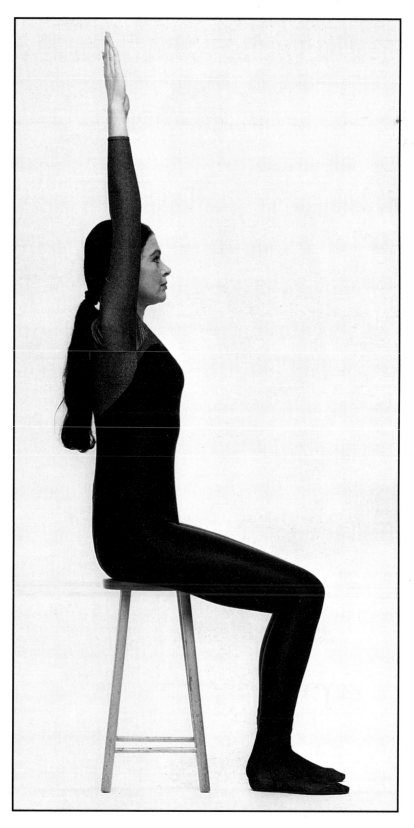

Slowly bring your hands up stretched and in front of you, and stretch them above your head up by the sides of your ears and reach for the ceiling – really stretch! Bring your arms slowly down on to your knees and relax. Repeat six times. Aim to take one minute.

Neck Rolling

Sit perfectly straight so that you can feel that your neck and shoulders are completely free and that there is a general relaxed feeling.

Then slowly start to roll your head. First drop your head on to your chest.

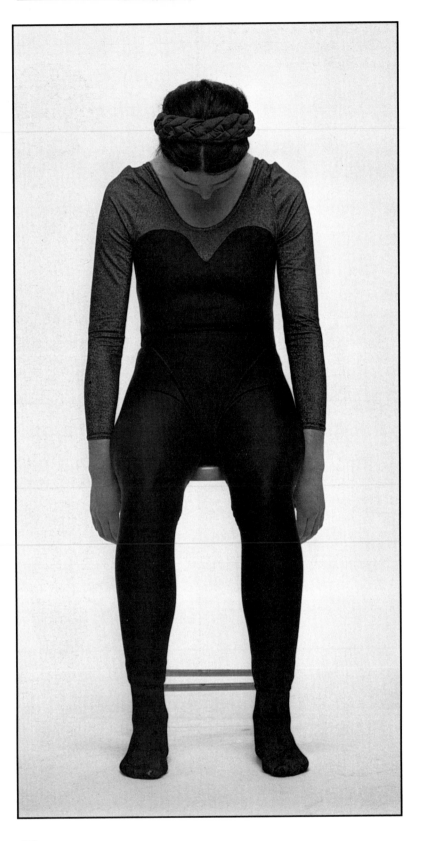

Then slowly swing your head into a rolling motion, bringing it slowly up by the right shoulder.

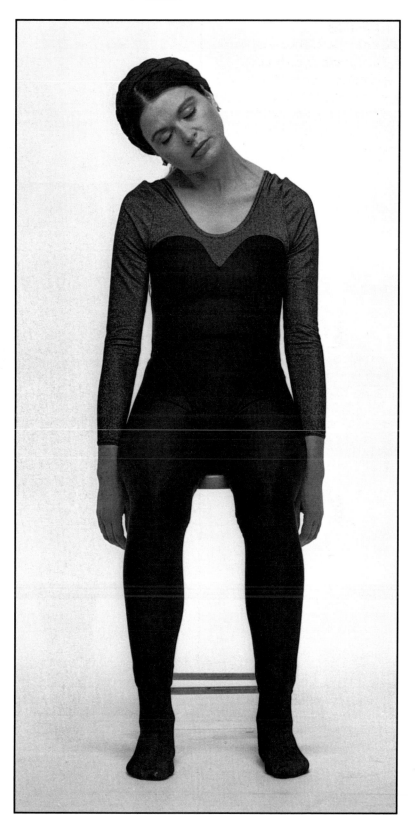

Let your head drop back.

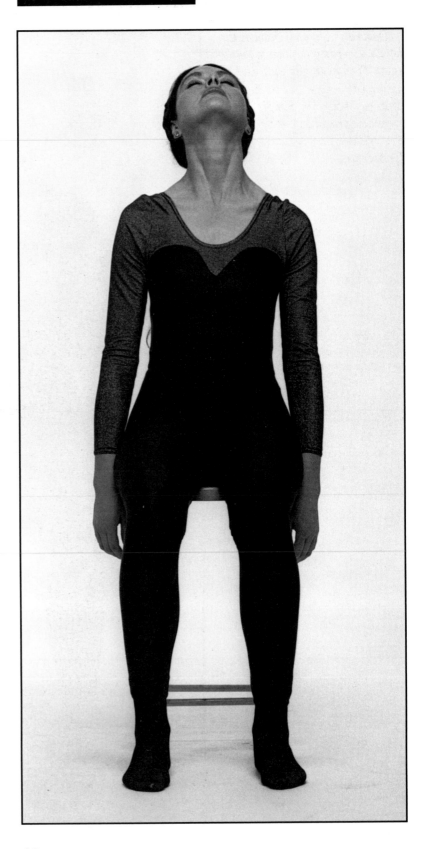

Then roll right over down by the left shoulder and back on to the chest. Then go the opposite way again. Do this exercise six times each way then relax. Simply let your shoulders drop away from you – that is the feeling you want. Do this for one minute.

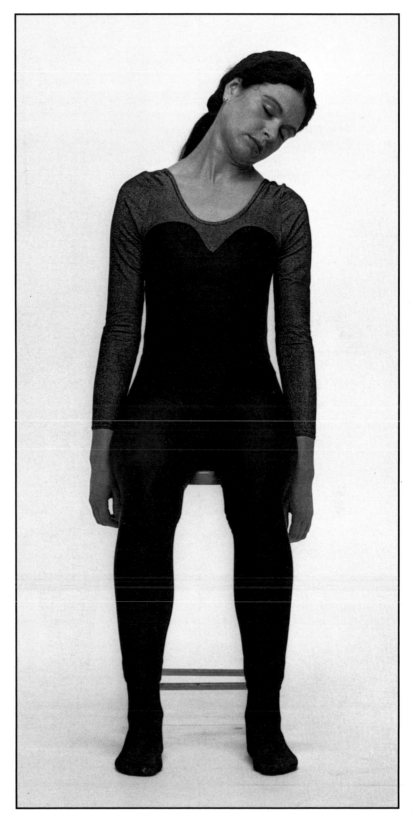

Posture Exercise
Still sitting on a stool, stretch your
arms as far behind you as possible,
then place left fist into the right
palm and push back as strenuously
as possible. Relax and bring hands
back to your behind. Repeat that
position six times and then place

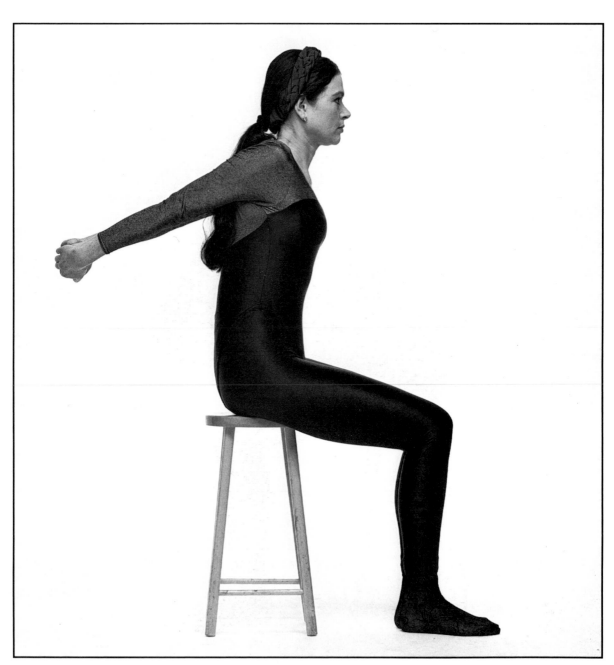

30

right fist into the left palm. Again, do the exercise six times, then relax. Breathe in as you push the hands out and breathe out as you relax.

A wonderful exercise for posture. Again, perform this exercise for one minute.

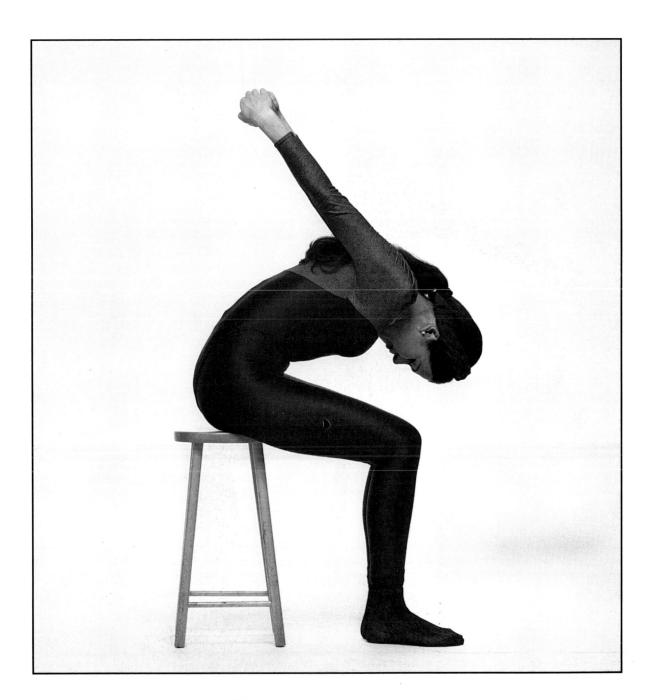

PRESSURE POINT MASSAGING

Most of you will already know the 15 pressure point programme that follows. For those of you who don't, there are full instructions. Check and double check you have the correct position for each pressure point.

Most beginnners do not massage with enough vigour. Press as hard as you can without hurting yourself. This is not just a spiritual exercise. Remember, you are dispersing the toxins on your terminal nerve endings.

But do concentrate too on the spiritual side of things. As you massage each pressure point, visualize to yourself the benefits described, so that the sub-conscious power of your mind will concentrate your body's regenerative energy to the best end. See in your mind's eye, for instance, how massaging the pressure point connected with the liver clears your skin, how massaging the point for the sex glands gives you that extra sparkle in your eyes, and how massaging your thyroids helps you to achieve your correct weight. In this way your pressure point massage becomes twice as effective.

In addition, I am going to show you how to massage some extra pressure points – the ones on your skull. This will tone up your whole body, giving you a feeling of a rush of energy to the head, and it will relieve any lingering tension there.

And lastly, I am going to teach you the magic of the Abdominal-Lock Exercise. This is a secret I learned from monks in the Himalayas, most of whom live to be over a hundred. Legend has it that there, practice of this exercise makes the old become young again. When I returned home, my research showed that this abdominal-lock exercise has a scientific basis in Zone Therapy. It is unique in that it is the only exercise in the Zone Therapy system that enables us to exercise our glands and organs directly. It has a fantastic effect on the central nervous system, the sympathetic nervous system and the cerebral spinal nervous system.

It will awaken you to powers that have been dormant for so long, you will see things in a different light and, in the words of the monks, receive many blessings.

THE TECHNIQUES OF TOUCHING

Spend thirty seconds on each pressure point, that is a total of seven minutes on this fifteen point programme. As I have said, we all have an instinctive need to care for and heal ourselves by touch, but we don't know exactly how or where. This is what I am now going to teach you. The zones of the body vary slightly in position in each individual so the pressure points I give you in the charts and in the text and photographs are approximate. If you don't find it exactly as in the chart and photograph, either go slightly below, slightly above, or to the side and you will contact the right point; you will be able to tell when you have done this because the exact spot for you will be the one that is sore and sensitive – this is because of the toxins you have accumulated there.

Make certain that your nails are cut short so that you don't lacerate your skin. Use the top joint of the thumb. Place the top of the thumb over the point indicated in the diagram and press into the area, rotating in a clockwise motion or anti-clockwise motion, whichever you like, as long as you remember to use a rotating movement. You can use the fingertips in the same way.

Always massage with an upward and outward circular movement. Remember you are breaking down the toxins blocking your nerve endings to allow energy, blood and oxygen to reach your face. You can work quite deeply on the various pressure points with a very firm action. (The exceptions are pressure points 3, 4 and 15, where you must use a more gentle massage movement.)

Some people can take more pressure than others. For all points apart from 3, 4 and 15, press *as hard as you can* without feeling uncomfortable. You will find your own level by what you feel. Where there is deep congestion it will be tender and you will be able to bear less pressure to begin with, so use your common sense and don't work at it too vigorously. Over a period of time you will be able to massage more deeply as you remove the condition. And after a series of treatments you will break down the crystaline deposits and completely free all the systems, enabling them to return to normal activity.

I repeat: do not apply consistent pressure for long periods over hurtful spots. Give painful areas a few seconds' pressure, then move on and come back to the tender places after a short rest.

In fact Zone Therapy is usually quite painful in many areas in the beginning but, over a period of time, as you eliminate poison from the particular nerve ending and stimulate the gland, the painful areas will decrease, until eventually there is no tenderness left in that particular area. When you have done that, you know you have done a good job!

It doesn't matter at what time of day you carry out the treatment, but it is important to do it regularly. Just imagine: in ten minutes, as well as giving your complexion the attention it surely deserves, you have helped to tone up your entire system.

Now we will go on to the VITAL PRESSURE POINTS on your face to get your face and body under your control.

How to massage your face
*Refer to the face chart and
accompanying photographs, and
start to work on each pressure point
in turn, beginning with number 1
and continuing to number 15.
Spend thirty seconds on each
pressure point.*

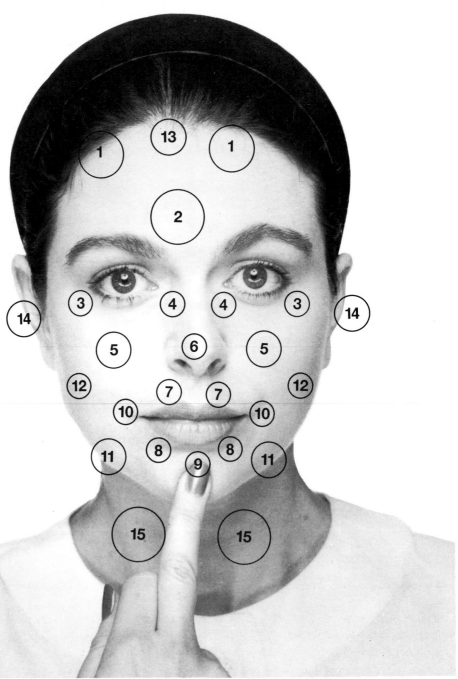

34

1 MENTAL STIMULATION

CLEAR THE MIND AND PURIFY THE SKIN

Surprisingly enough, massaging these areas can actually improve your thinking processes and activate your reflexes. The pressure you exert also clears blockages in the nerve endings in the forehead, allowing more blood and oxygen to reach your skin and so purifying your face.

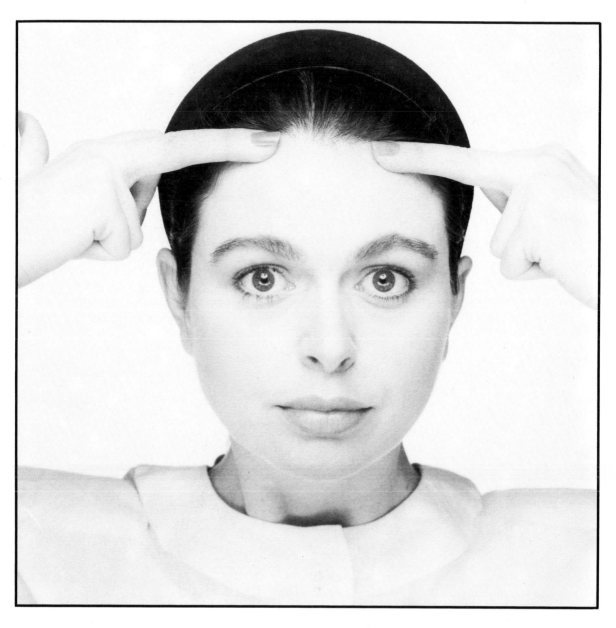

Find the edge of the forehead, where the bone indents, then with a firm upward and outward circular movement of about half-an-inch radius move slowly with both fingers in towards the centre of the forehead, then out again. Complete four times. Remember, if it is tender, that is because poisons are blocking the proper functioning of this zone in your body.

2 THE PITUITARY GLAND AND THIRD EYE

BRING ALL YOUR GLANDS INTO PERFECT BALANCE

Pressure here stimulates the pituitary gland. This produces the hormones needed by the entire reproductive system. It is the master gland and should be kept in perfect working order. You will find to your astonishment that massaging this area will enliven your imagination and greatly improve your perception.

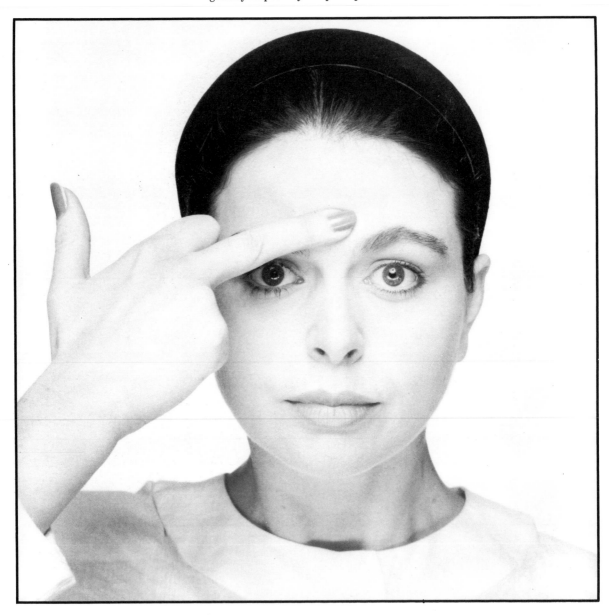

Find the slight indent in your forehead. Massage again, upward and outward in a half-inch radius for thirty seconds.

3 THE COLONS

REDUCE PUFFINESS AND BLOTCHINESS IN THE SKIN

It is vital to keep the colons in good working order. If they begin to malfunction, poisons will build up internally because waste matter is not being eliminated properly. The appearance of the face will suffer accordingly.

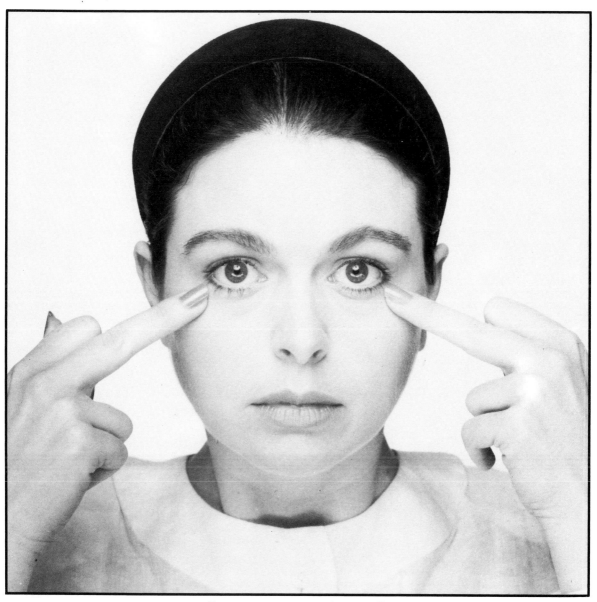

To massage pressure points 3 and 4, tap gently underneath the eye, starting on the outside and moving inwards towards the nose, then out again. Complete four times.

37

4 KIDNEY STIMULATION

CLEAN YOUR BLOOD AND THEREFORE YOUR SKIN OF ALL
IMPURITIES

Healthy kidneys eliminate toxins and acidity. As most of the food we eat
has a good deal of acidity, it is easy to see how vital these organs are.
Any abnormality will affect a person's general health and the skin on
the face will suffer very badly.

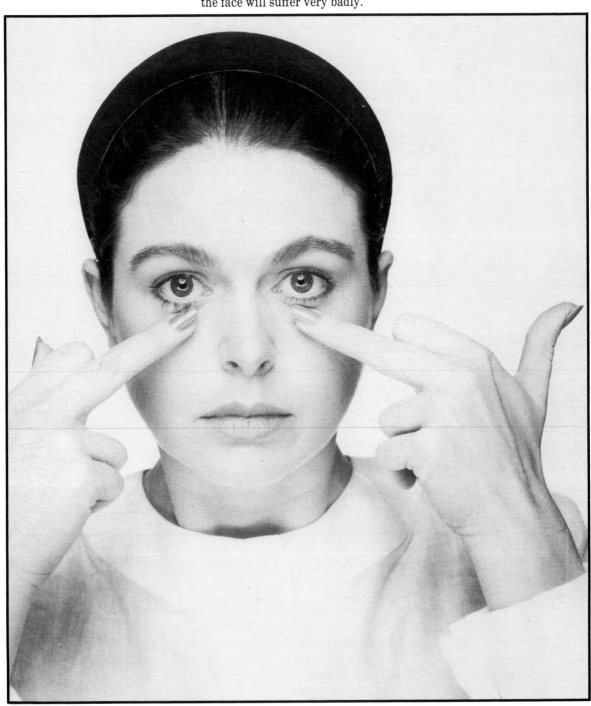

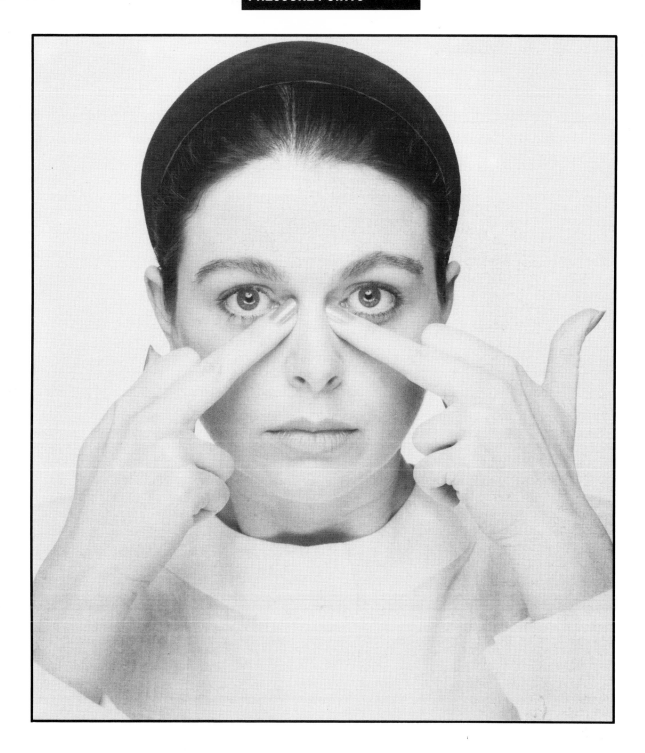

5 HEALTHY BOWEL ACTION

MAKE YOUR SKIN LUSTROUS

Most of us don't think too much about our bowels. We should. Sluggish bowels are one of the main reasons for dull-looking, pasty skin. Massage the appropriate pressure points well.

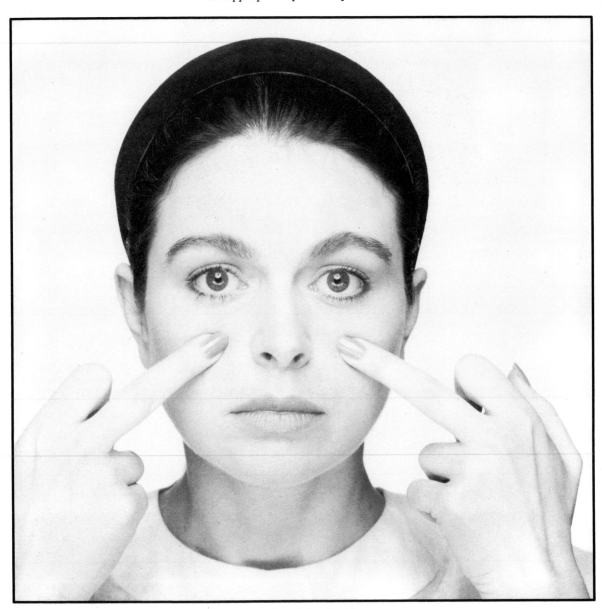

Find the ridge of the cheekbone at its highest point, then press up into it, then massage as hard as you can in an upward and outward circular movement, while moving slowly the length of the cheekbone. Complete four times.

6 STOMACH PROBLEMS

IMPROVE AND EVEN OUT SKIN TONE

Sufferers from digestive trouble may be surprised to learn that simply by massaging the tip of the nose vigorously, their digestion will be greatly improved. It's all to do with blocked nerve endings again.

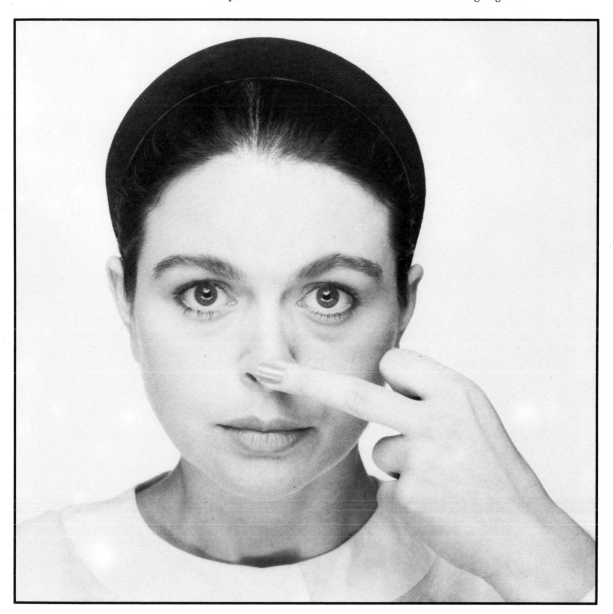

Without lifting the fingers, slide along the skin of your nose, press as hard as you feel comfortable with and rotate slowly for thirty seconds.

7 THE SPLEEN

ENERGIZE YOUR WHOLE FACE
A healthy spleen means a healthy stomach, so be sure to massage these areas thoroughly.

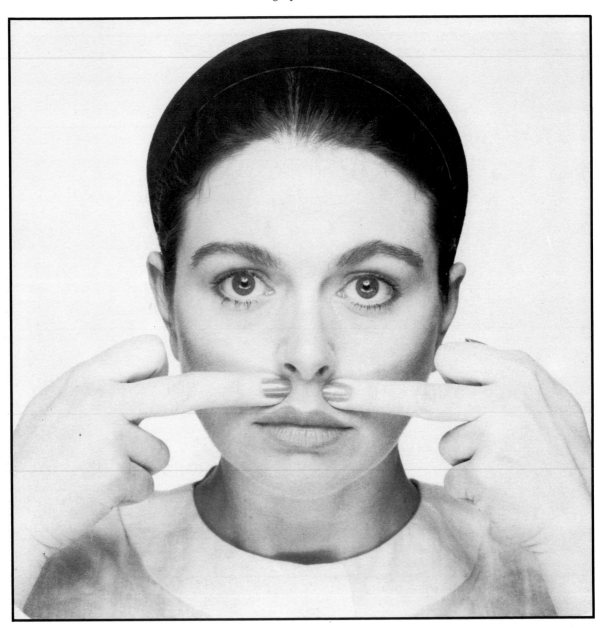

Pressing inwards on either side of the ridge that runs from your nose to the middle of your upper lip, rotate your fingers in a half-inch radius. Press hard so that you feel your gums underneath.

8 PANCREAS

PURIFY THE SKIN

This secretes alkaline enzymes which help the digestive process. A malfunction can cause too much acidity which is very harmful to the skin. So massaging these areas thoroughly can help to attain a beautiful skin and face.

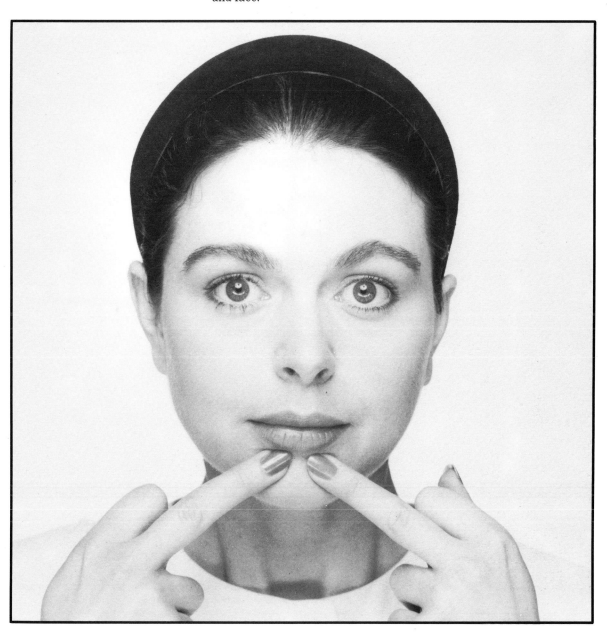

Starting at the extremities of the underside of the lips, work inwards with a firm rotating motion towards the centre, then out again. Complete four times. Feel your lower gums through your lower lip.

9 BOWELS

ELIMINATE TOXINS FROM THE SKIN

Sufferers from constipation will not need to be reminded what a problem it is. It's one of the main causes of sluggishness and lack of energy. A build-up of large amounts of toxins result in lacklustre skin and eyes and unpleasant breath. Vigorous massaging of this area will greatly help to rectify the condition and bring back life and colour to the face.

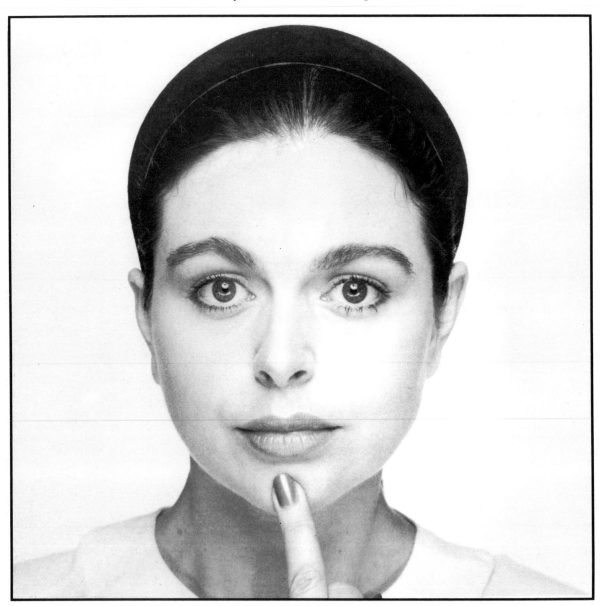

Find the indent in your chin, then rotate as firmly as you can bear for thirty seconds.

10 LUNGS

PUT POWER INTO YOUR FACE

Massaging this area will persuade the lungs to work better, helping to keep colds, bronchitis and asthma at bay. The better supply of oxygen resulting will improve not only the skin of the face but that of the whole body.

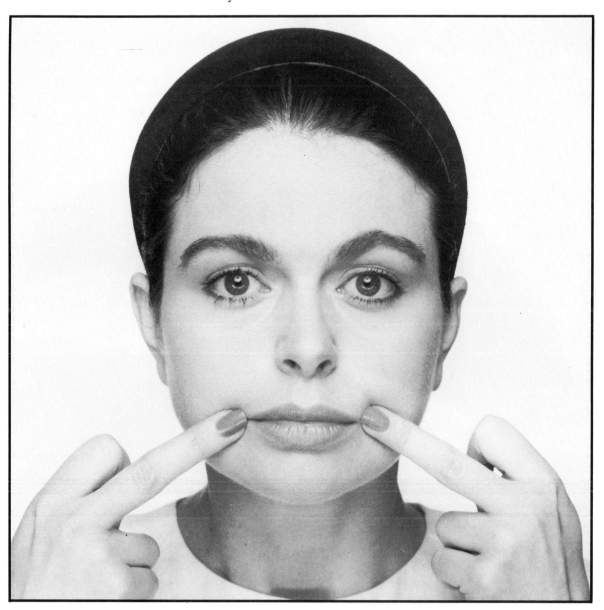

Find the muscle running down the length of the side of the mouth, then press inwards and outward with your rotating motion as hard as you can bear for thirty seconds.

11 SEXUAL DESIRE

INCREASE SEXUAL ATTRACTION
The health of the sex glands is important to all of us. Their failure can bring impotence, lack of sex drive and lack of control. So it is advisable to massage these areas vigorously as they affect the entire reproductive system. The proper functioning of the sex glands brings a glow to face and skin.

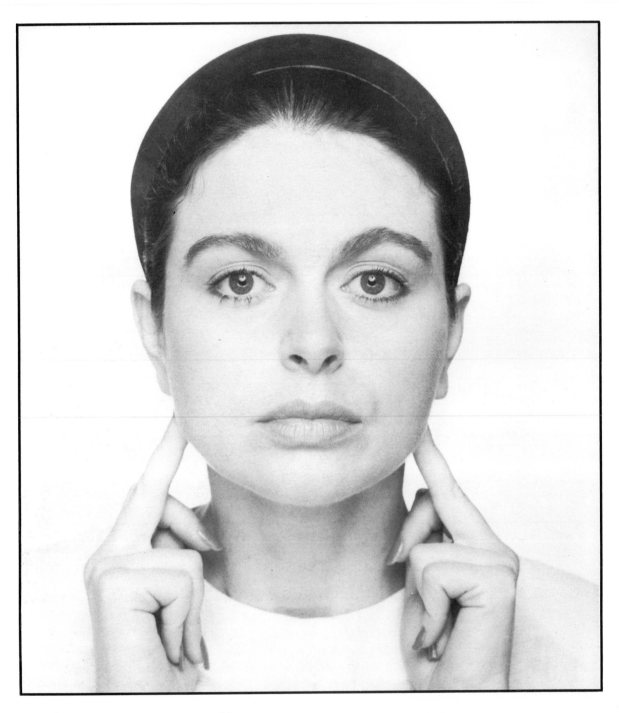

12 THE LIVER AND LYMPHATIC SYSTEM

ELIMINATE EXCESS FLUID AND REDUCE WEIGHT

For us to feel truly well and look really healthy it is vital to keep the liver in peak condition. A sluggish liver affects the entire body, especially the facial skin. The liver helps to purify the blood; impure blood means sagging skin and a face that looks older than it should. Massage in these areas also tones up the lymphatic system which is important to general health and to a lovely face and skin.

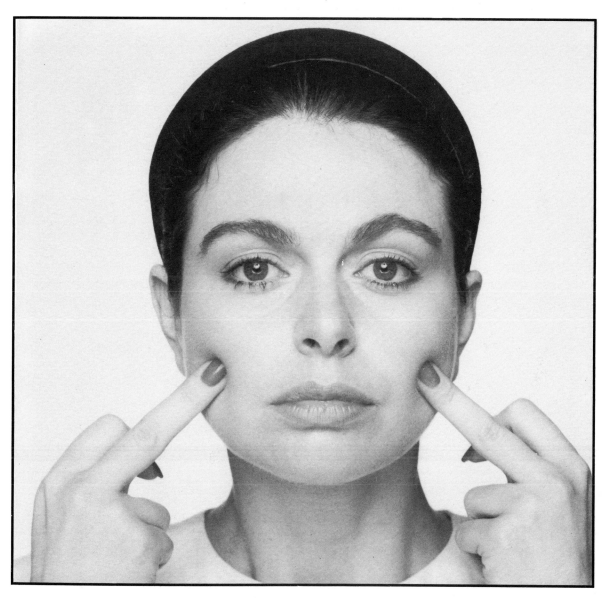

◀ *Starting immediately below the ear, rub with your rotating movement along the ridge of the jawbone until you are directly underneath the pupils of your eyes. Work back again and repeat four times as hard as you can.*

Find the deepest pit of the cheek, where the jawbone meets the cheekbones. Work in a half-inch radius as hard as you can for thirty seconds.

47

13 SYMPATHETIC NERVOUS SYSTEM

REMOVE WORRY LINES

Massaging this area tones up the whole nervous system and brings a sense of peace and tranquillity. This feeling of well-being is always reflected in the face.

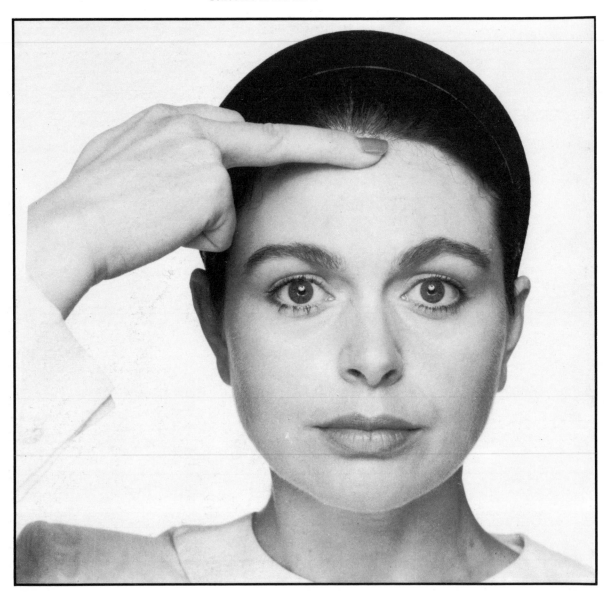

Work the centre point high on your forehead in a half-inch radius as hard as you can for thirty seconds.

14 TONING UP THE ENTIRE BODY

IMPROVE FACIAL MUSCLES AND YOUR ENTIRE SYSTEM
Massage both ears in turn by taking the entire ear between fingers and thumb. Start at the top and work up and down as hard as you can four times. After a few minutes your whole system will be pervaded by a glowing tingle. The effect will be seen in the facial muscles and the general tone of the face.

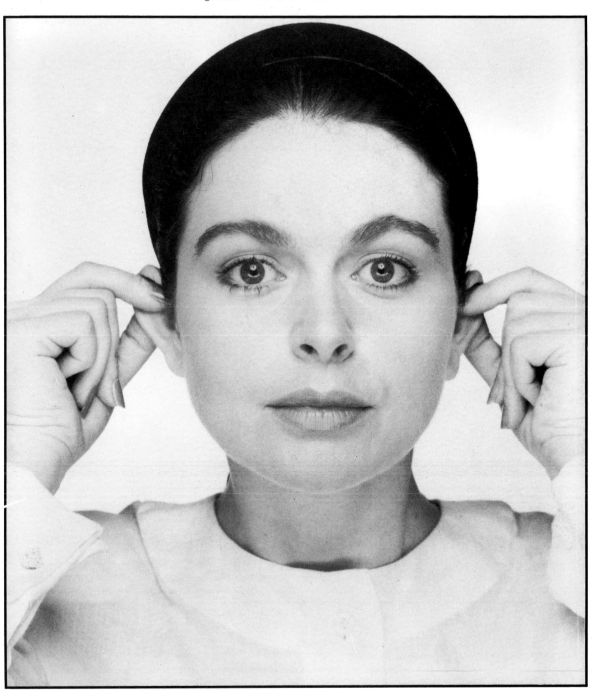

15 THE THYROIDS

HELPING YOU TO ACHIEVE YOUR IDEAL WEIGHT

The thyroids are situated on either side of the windpipe. They are vital to good health for, if they fail to work properly, the body becomes sluggish, the heartbeat is lowered and breathing becomes laboured. Sufferers feel the cold intensely and may put on weight; their circulation is poor and their skin becomes dry and scaly. They may also be distressed and unhappy and suffer several other unwanted symptoms including poor memory and problems with menstruation. All this from the two little glands.

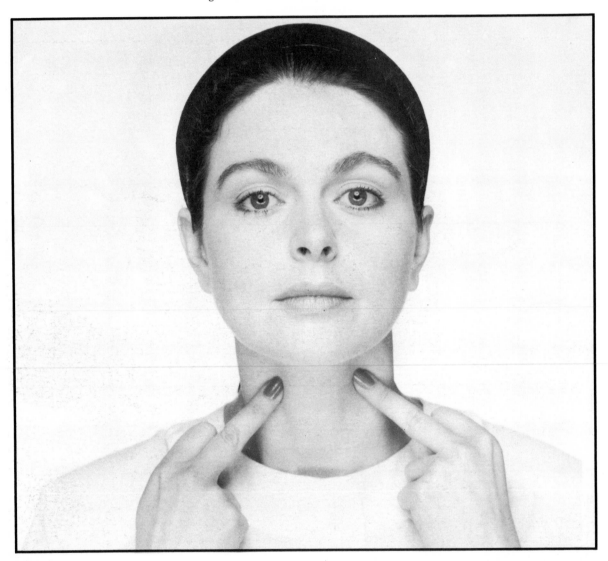

To avoid all these ills and enjoy beautiful skin, work gently but well over the thyroid glands. Starting either side of the thyroids, move inwards and upwards with a gentle circular movement. Complete four times.

THE SCALP MASSAGE
At the high point of your neck at the back, at the indentation where the neck meets the skull, there is an important pressure point. By massaging it for thirty seconds you can get rid of tension – including many headaches – and empty the lymph gland by which the body stores excess liquid.

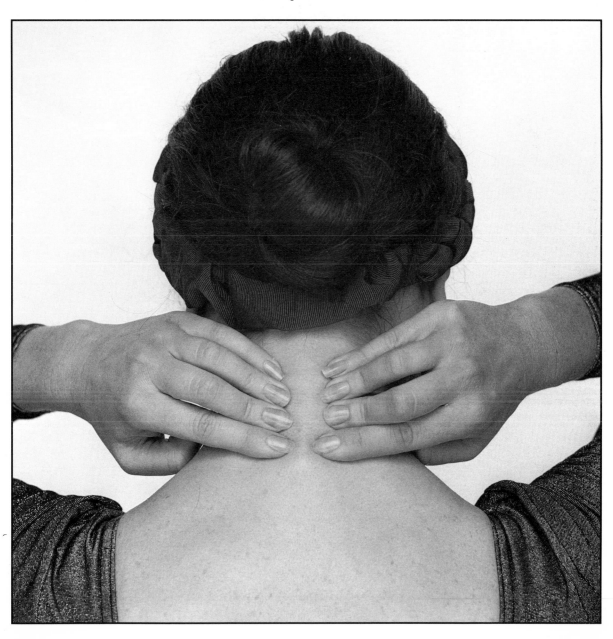

Perform this massage for a count of twenty, then, without removing your fingers from the surface of your head, continue to massage in small circles working out to the tendons on either side; then move gradually up your tendons and over the top of your scalp – your fingers should

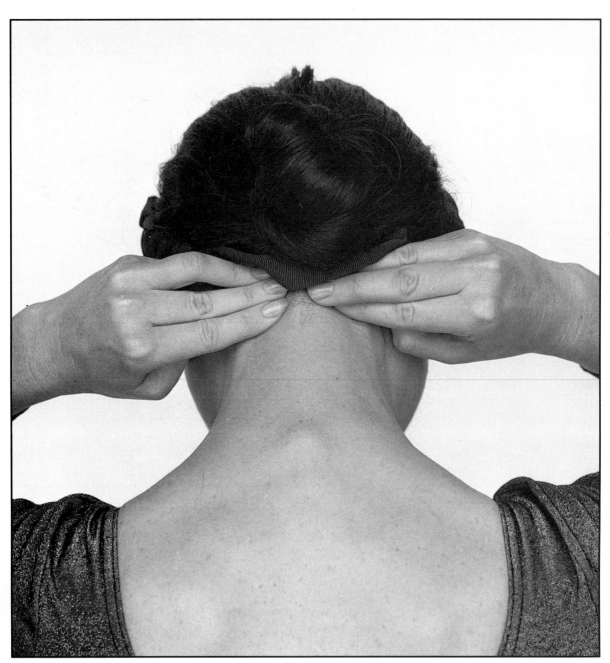

*remain in parallel about 2 inches
apart – the same distance as the gap
between your tendons – until you
reach the hair-line at the front.*

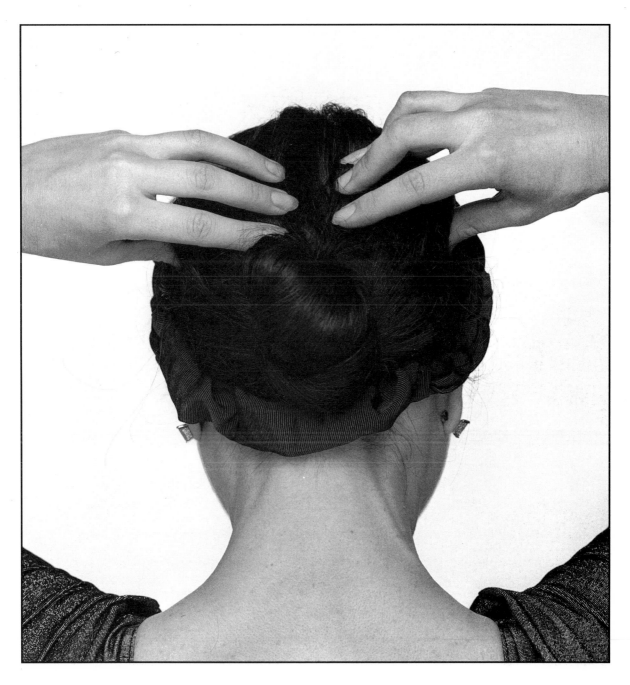

Next move slowly along the hair-line to just above and behind the ears. This massage takes a total of one and a half minutes.

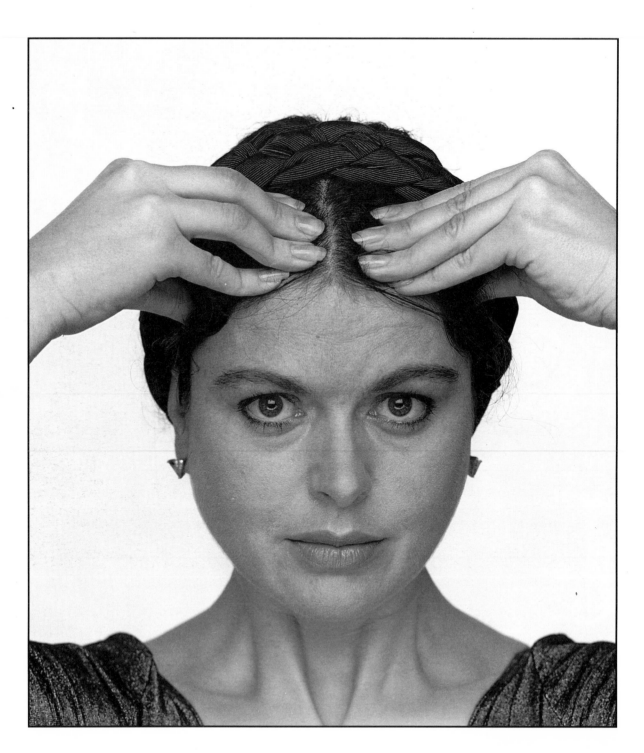

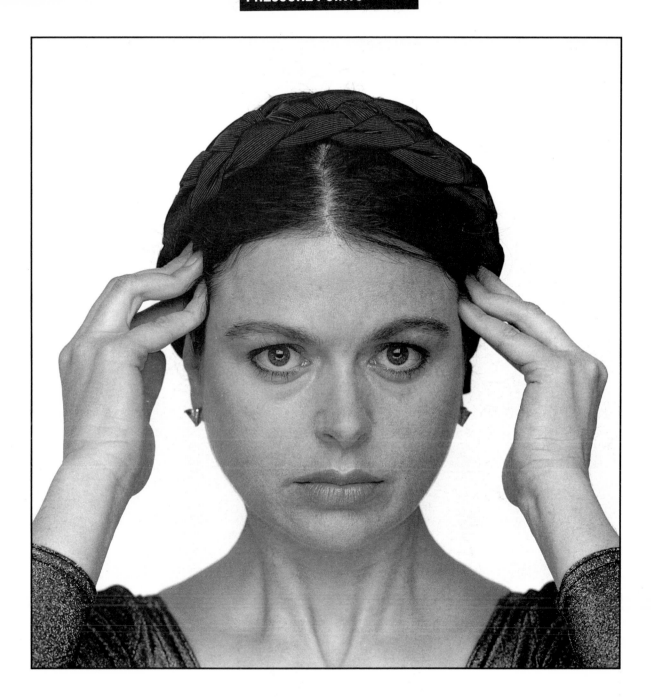

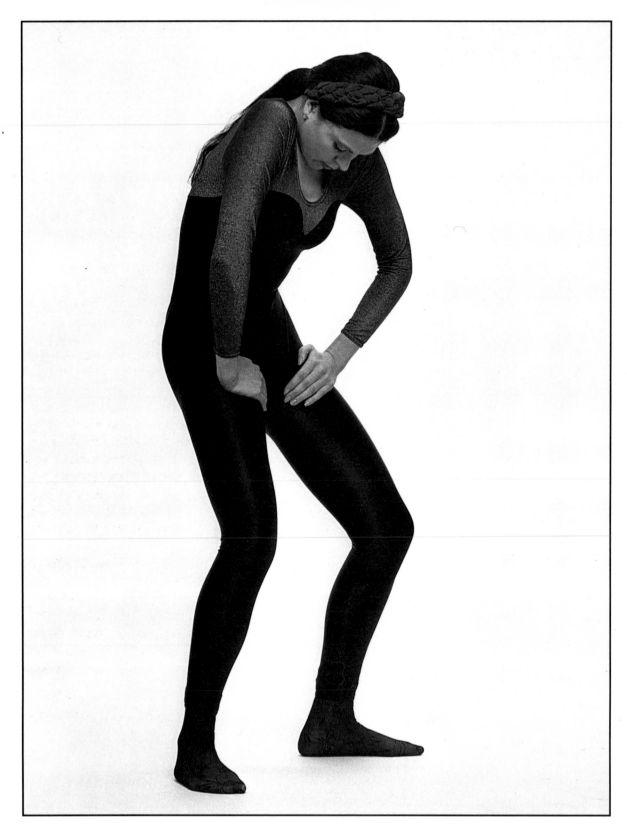

THE ABDOMINAL-LOCK EXERCISE

It is said in the East that the practiser of this exercise, if old, becomes young again.

A detailed description will make it easy to learn. Stand with the feet apart and hands on the bent legs in a semi-squatting position.

Make yourself comfortable in the posture and then empty the lungs forcing the breath out. Contract the abdominal muscles. Raise the viscera until a large depression is made under the diaphragm, for a count of ten. One should be able to place both fists in the pocket that is made. Then suddenly relax.

Repeat this alternating contraction and relaxation three times before taking another breath. Practise and soon you will be doing it for five counts. Continue practising until you can do it for ten counts. Before the next round stand up straight and rest for a few seconds until the flow of breath returns.

When you have rested, empty your lungs and repeat the process. The average individual should be able to do five rounds.

Never force any exercise or impose a strain upon the system. If this exercise causes undue fatigue, stop immediately. The practice of these exercises is designed to make you grow strong and this requires time. Naturally this will vary for each individual depending on age, physical structure and condition at the time of starting the practice. Do not sacrifice the vigour of contraction for speed which will come in due time.

It was not long before I could execute twenty contractions on each exhalation for ten rounds. I kept this pace up for one month. After my muscles became hard I practised every morning and late in the afternoon before dinner. After another month I added five rounds each week to my daily schedule until I reached five hundred contractions for each session.

After one has a measure of one's capacity and has accustomed the body to the exercise, it is possible to increase the number of strokes for each exhalation. My final goal was 750 contractions. This was over a period of two years.

You must start with a count of three, and if you master ten strokes on each exhalation, then you are doing pretty well.

If you are in normal health the exercise will, without a shadow of doubt, go almost 100 per cent to making sure that all the internal parts of your body in that particular region function perfectly. Practise it for just one and a half minutes a day.

You have just done yourself more good in these last ten minutes than you will do for yourself the rest of the day.

You are one large step nearer being more youthful, more beautiful and more healthy than you could have ever imagined.

You have just opened up the channels of the body's natural regenerating power by pressure point massage. We are now going to concentrate on using this power to rebuild your muscles.

Muscle wastage, as I say, causes people to age most visibly, most quickly. As your muscles slacken, lengthen and thin out, your skin becomes looser and saggier and more wrinkly. But, spend ten minutes every day performing the following face-building exercises, and your skin will become as tight as any surgical facelift can make it. Not, however, in an artificial way: your muscles will cling energetically to the bone and pulse with life, so that the skin attached to them is pulled up and clear and firm, rippling with youth, beauty and health.

After only a few weeks you will see a radical difference. You will begin to look the way you did years ago.

Again, I must emphasize that it is important to practise these exercises with as much vigour as possible. When you are asked to stretch a particular muscle, concentrate only on that muscle, stretching it as far as you can. The rest of your face should be totally relaxed from the relaxation exercises we practised a few minutes ago. So, too, when you are asked to push with your muscle against your hands or fingers, push as hard as you can, concentrating only on that muscle and feeling the muscle resistance.

These stretching and pushing exercises employ the basic principles used by body-builders. Pressure and resistance is what builds muscle. There is no other way. In the case of the face it is impossible to over-build your muscles. Practise the following exercises daily in conjunction with your pressure point massage and aim to look twenty-five again. And, as I say, if you are twenty-five or younger, practise these exercises and this massage and you need never grow old.

You must practise each of these exercises as vigorously as you can for just thirty seconds each. Aim to complete the course in approximately ten minutes. You will find it extremely tough at first; but just concentrate on performing as many exercises as you can within the ten minutes. Try to improve day by day, performing more of the exercises within these ten minutes. Even after your first attempt, you will feel the power of renewed youth oozing up and into your face. Your face will feel more alive than you can ever remember it feeling.

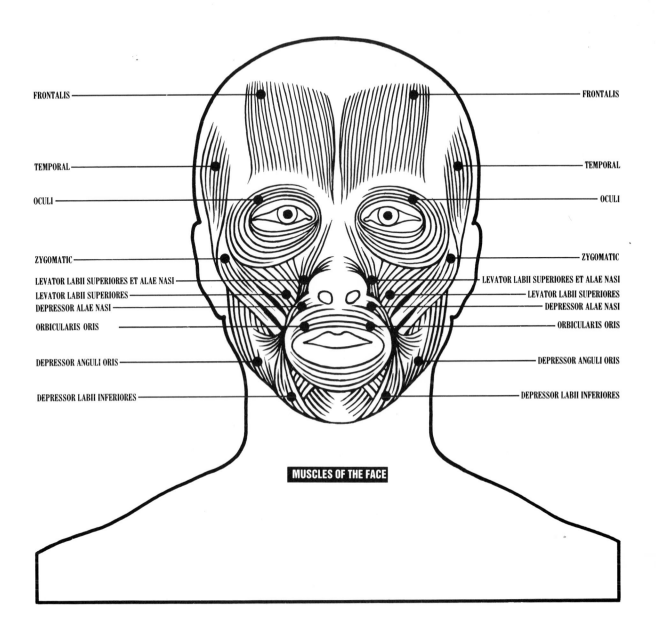

FRONTALIS

TEMPORAL

OCULI

ZYGOMATIC

LEVATOR LABII SUPERIORES ET ALAE NASI

LEVATOR LABII SUPERIORES

DEPRESSOR ALAE NASI

ORBICULARIS ORIS

DEPRESSOR ANGULI ORIS

DEPRESSOR LABII INFERIORES

FRONTALIS

TEMPORAL

OCULI

ZYGOMATIC

LEVATOR LABII SUPERIORES ET ALAE NASI

LEVATOR LABII SUPERIORES

DEPRESSOR ALAE NASI

ORBICULARIS ORIS

DEPRESSOR ANGULI ORIS

DEPRESSOR LABII INFERIORES

MUSCLES OF THE FACE

FACE EXERCISES

Exercise one

Sit on a chair as in the posture exercises, your face completely relaxed. Say the word 'Cue'; your lips will come forward, push your lips as far forward as possible – feel the muscle being worked.

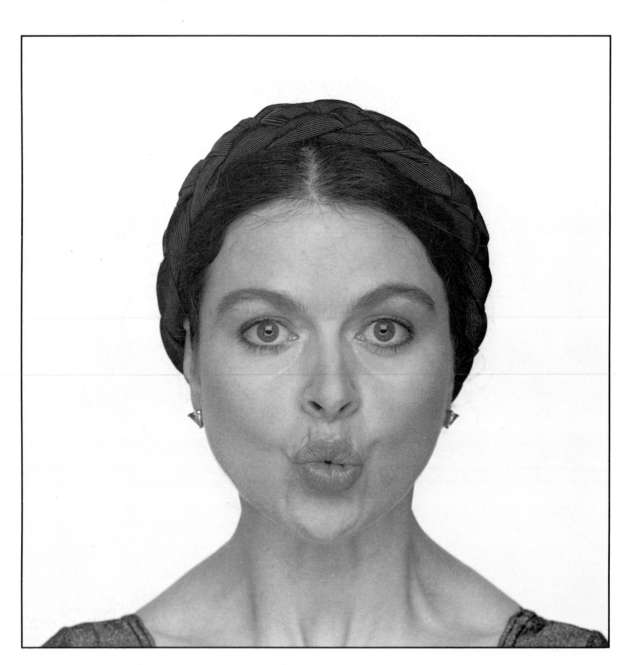

From that position open your mouth wide and say the word 'Ex', and pull back the muscles of your face as far as you can towards your ears. Try it slowly a couple of times to get the feel, and then do it quickly just thinking the words 'Cue' and 'Ex'. Repeat thirty times.

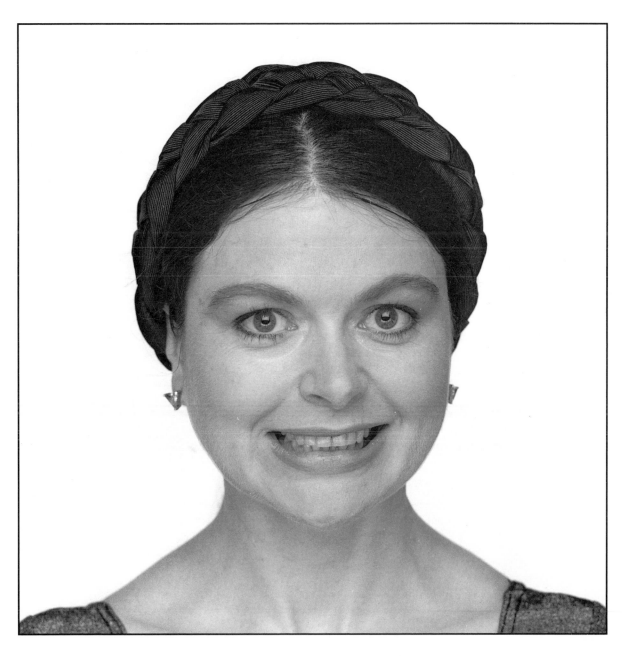

Exercise two

Open your mouth as wide as possible and stick your tongue out as far as possible. Open your eyes as wide as possible. You will feel all the muscles working. Try and do this exercise twenty times in thirty seconds. This is the way to make your facial muscles work – feel all those muscles in your face and neck responding to your workout.

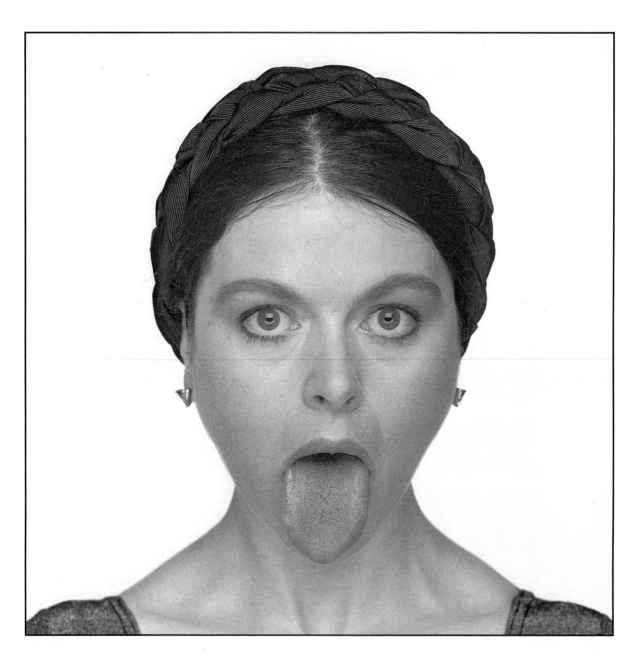

Exercise three

This is a beautiful smile but you are going to make each side of your mouth touch your ears. It's the kind of smile you see the clown in the circus do – an ear to ear smile. Try to touch your ears with the corners of your mouth and feel those muscles working. Put all your effort into it, holding three times for ten seconds each.

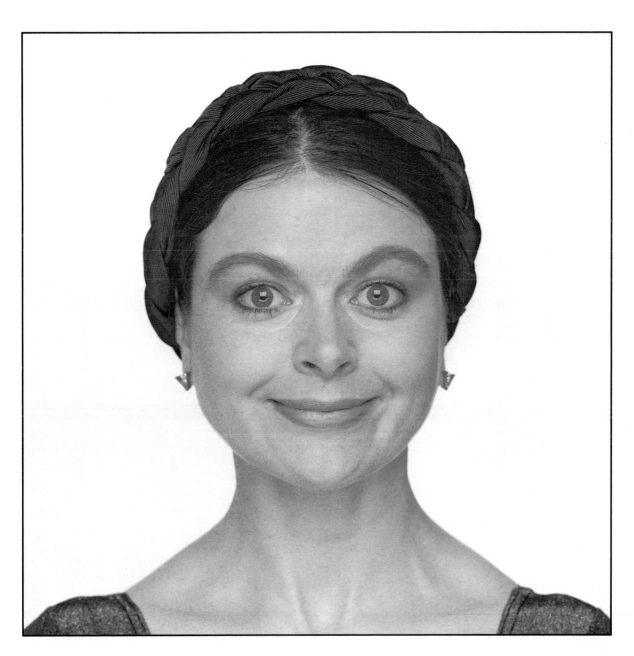

Exercise four

Close your eyes and pull a face as if you have smelled the most awful odour, the kind of face that says 'phew'. Then, open your eyes wide, at the same time opening your mouth wide enough to swallow an elephant. Try this exercise twenty times a day as quickly as you can, if possible within thirty seconds.

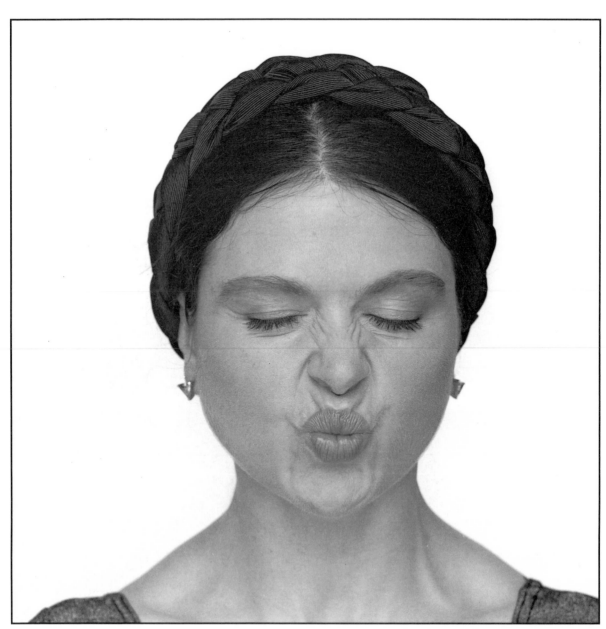

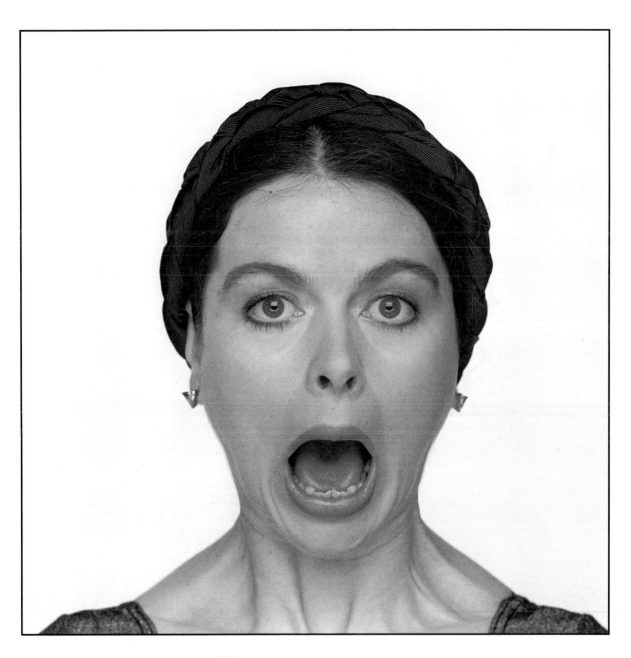

Exercise five

Purse your lips to the right and hold for five seconds, then purse to the left for five seconds. Do six, which will work out as three on each side of the face. So the exercise is done first to the right, then to the left. Do the exercises as quickly as possible. Put maximum effort into the

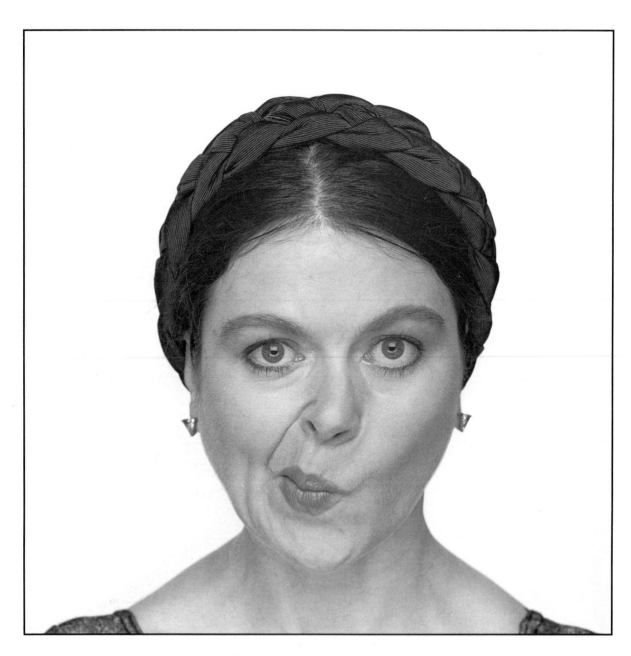

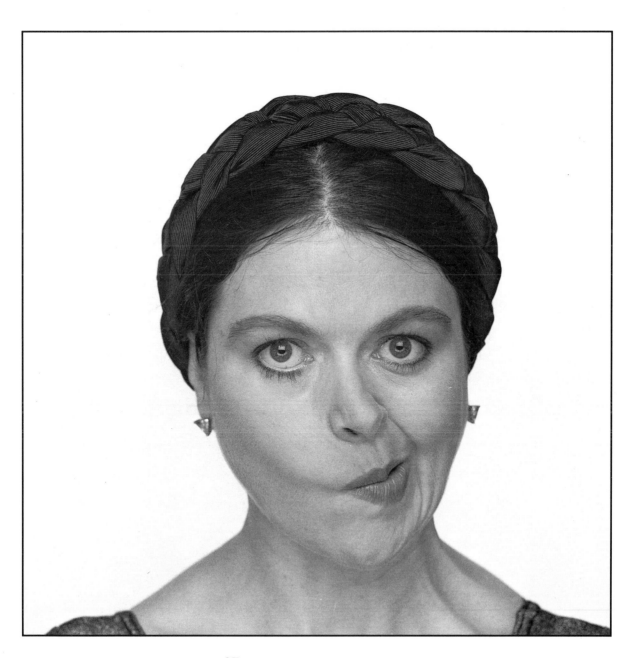

Exercise six
Study the photograph. Tilt the head
back, keeping teeth together, and
contract the neck and chin muscles.
Put your mind to it and make those
muscles work for thirty seconds.

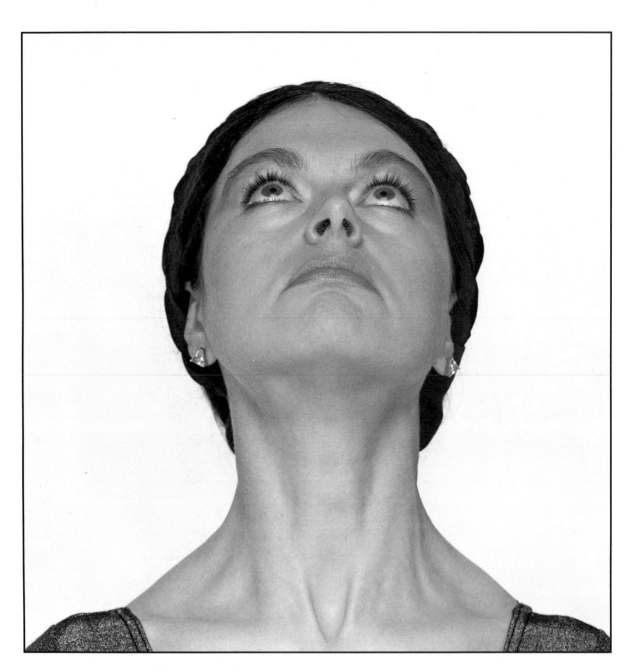

Exercise seven

Slightly separate teeth so that they are no longer in direct contact and do the previous exercise. Tilt the head slightly back and contract the throat and chin muscles. This will give your chin and·throat a terrific workout. Practice ten times per session.

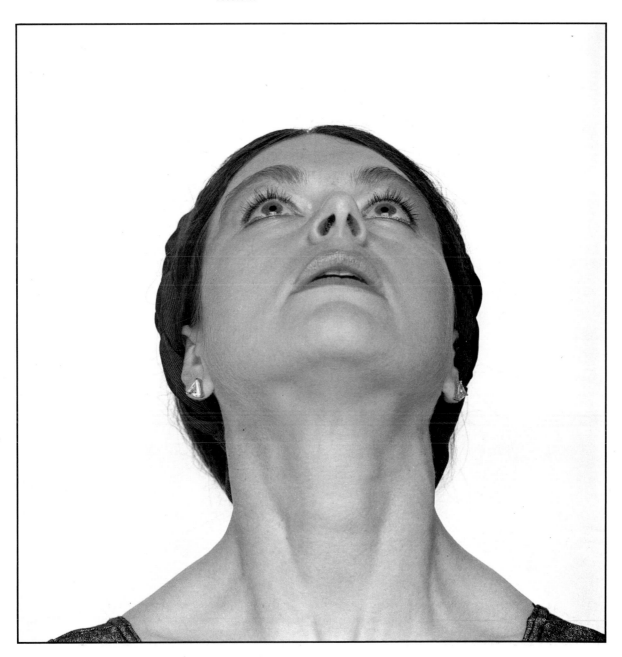

Exercise eight

Tilt your head slightly, lips together, teeth also together. Now, with the tip of your tongue, push your front top teeth as hard as you can, at the same time contracting the neck and chin muscles. Do this about ten times, then put the tip of your tongue against your bottom front teeth and push as hard as possible contracting the neck and chin muscles. Put your mind to it; you will find it is simply terrific. Feel the power of it. Do thirty contractions per session.

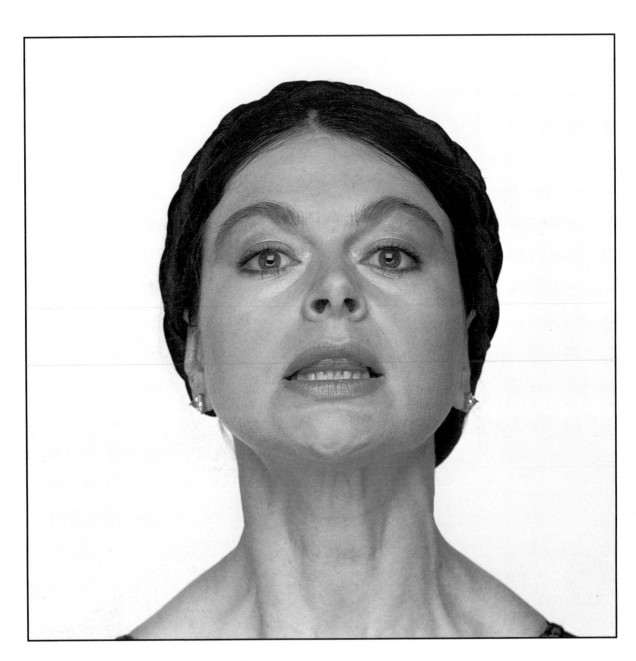

Exercise nine

This exercise is to help the cheek muscles which have lost the strength and power to hold their original line and position. If allowed to deteriorate, you will end up with lots of loose skin around the mouth and side of the chin. Slightly tilt your head. Bring your lower jaw and teeth as far forward as possible. Repeat this exercise twenty times. Then try to put your lower lip on to the tip of your nose. This is a powerful exercise for you to perform. Do this thirty times.

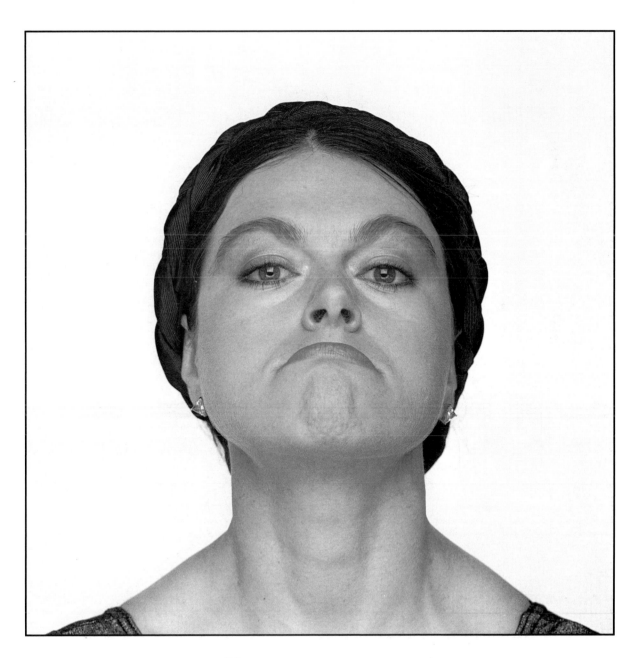

Exercise ten

Sit on a chair in front of a mirror, if possible; sit upright, relaxing face, neck and shoulders. Now close your eyes to a slit and contract the muscles under the eyes. Make sure the rest of the face is relaxed – only the muscles under the eyes must move. Put as much power as possible into the exercise. Hold for five seconds, and relax slowly, then contract the muscles again for five seconds. Do this exercise for thirty seconds.

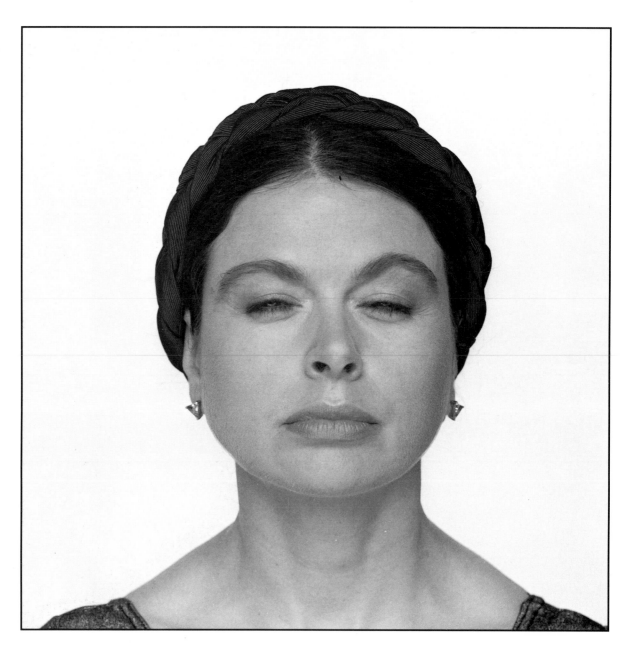

Exercise eleven

Your head, face, neck and shoulders should be relaxed. Now raise your eyebrows and contract the muscles under your eyes. Put your mind on to making the muscles under your eyes really work. Hold the contraction for five seconds, then relax. Do the exercise for thirty seconds.

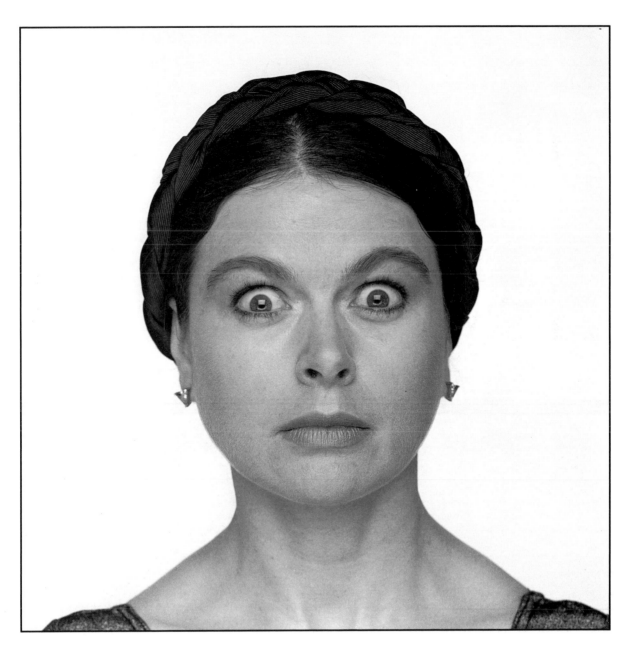

Exercise twelve

Try to keep your forehead in a relaxed state. Now place the thumb of your right hand under your right eyebrow and very firmly push upwards. Then concentrate on resisting with your mind focused on the spot where your thumb is. Put your will-power into lifting your eyebrow at the same time. Practise five-second contractions three times, then do the same with the left eyebrow.

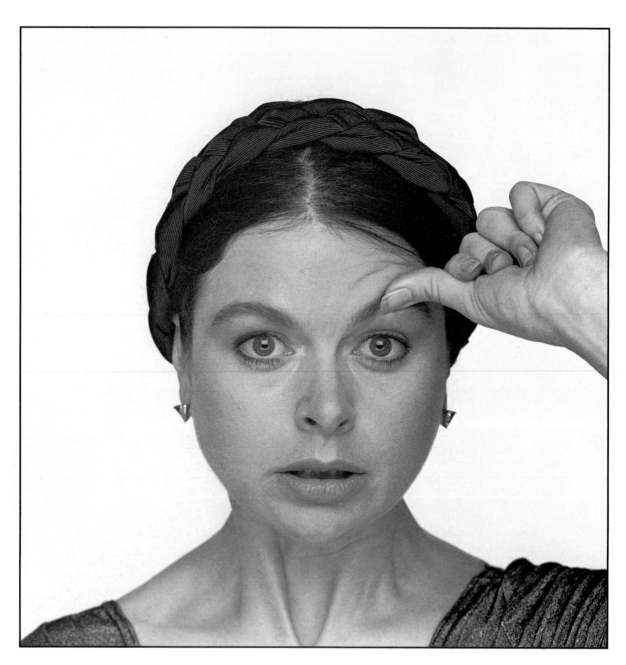

Exercise thirteen

With the thumb of your right hand still under your right eyebrow, try to close your right eye and at the same time imagine that your entire forehead is pressing down, forcing your eyebrow down and your eyelid to close. Practise a few times and you will begin to get the hang of it – it's not difficult, it just needs practice. After working on the right eyebrow, immediately do the same exercise on the left eyebrow. Spend fifteen seconds on each eyebrow.

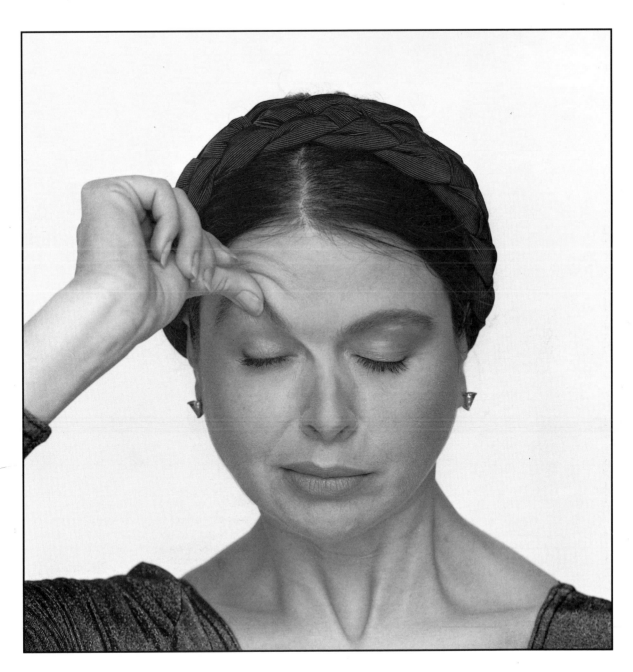

Exercise fourteen

For this exercise, close your eyes, concentrate on the muscles directly below your eyes, and contract them as strongly as possible. Do not frown or screw up your eyes, just close them and put power into the muscles underneath. Hold for five seconds, then slowly release. Spend thirty seconds on this exercise.

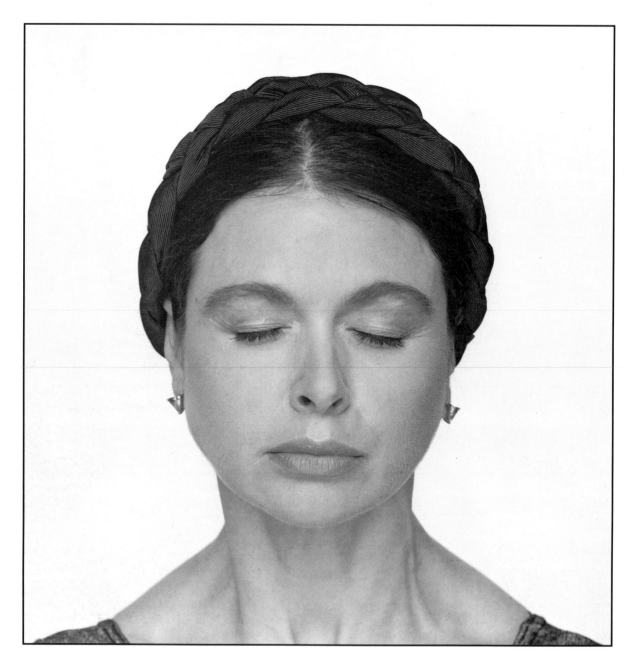

Exercise fifteen

Place the heels of the hands on the sides of the eyes as shown in the photo, then press firmly. Look upwards, face relaxed; now increase pressure at the sides of your eyes and raise your eyebrows as high as you can. Each time you raise your eyebrows, hold for a count of five seconds, then relax. Do not frown or wrinkle your forehead, just raise your eyebrows and put all your will-power and concentration into the exercise. Perform for thirty seconds.

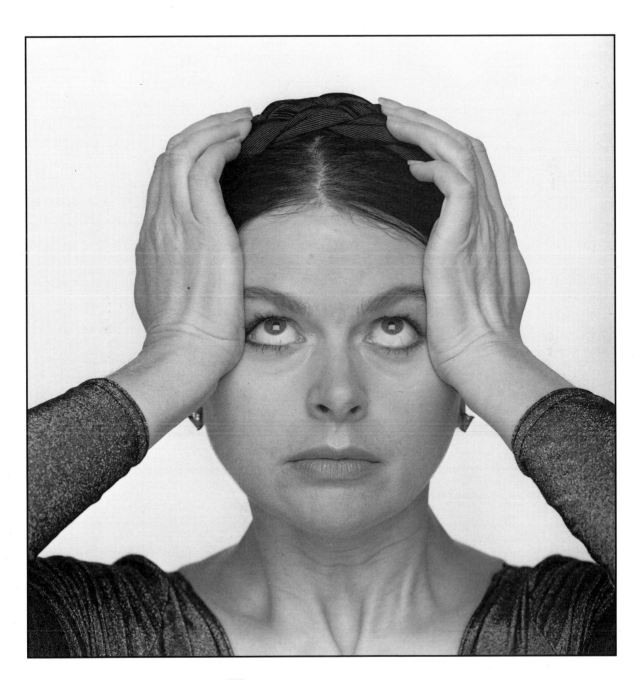

Exercise sixteen

Place both thumbs under the eyebrows, the right thumb under the right eyebrow and the left thumb under the left eyebrow. Push the eyebrows up with some force; at the same time, with all the will-power you can muster, try to close your eyelids. Hold for five seconds and relax for five seconds. Then repeat the exercise for thirty seconds.

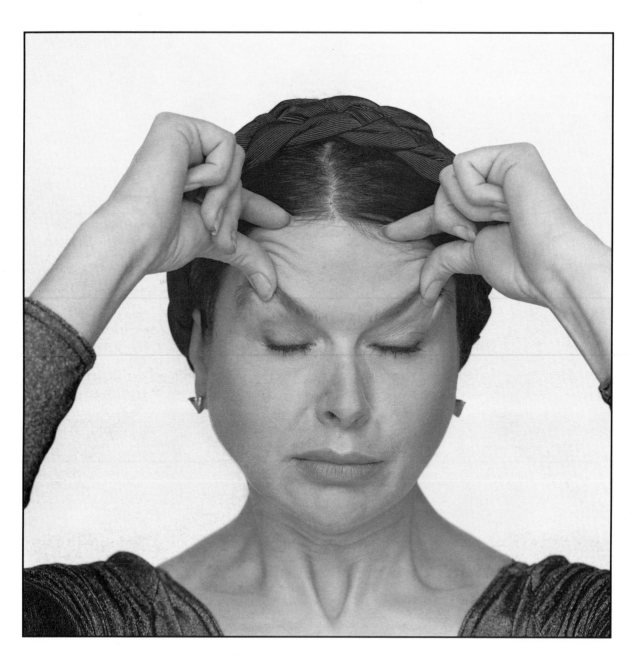

Exercise seventeen

Place the tip of the middle finger of both hands just above the bridge of the nose. Then add firm pressure towards the sides with the fingers, at the same time strongly resisting through the bridge of your nose with your will-power. Hold each pressure for five seconds. Do the exercise for thirty seconds and, above all, concentrate.

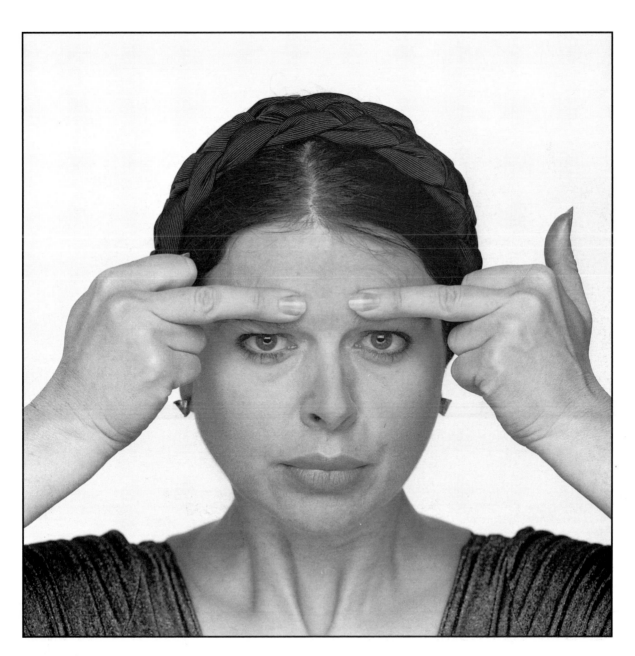

Exercise eighteen

Place the hands on the forehead as seen in the photo, putting on as much pressure as possible with your hand and fingers; whilst holding the pressure, apply your will-power and mind and try to move your entire forehead downwards. Close your eyes with each contraction and pull down. All this must come through your will-power. With a little bit of practice you will master the technique. Hold the contraction for five seconds at a time. Do this exercise for thirty seconds.

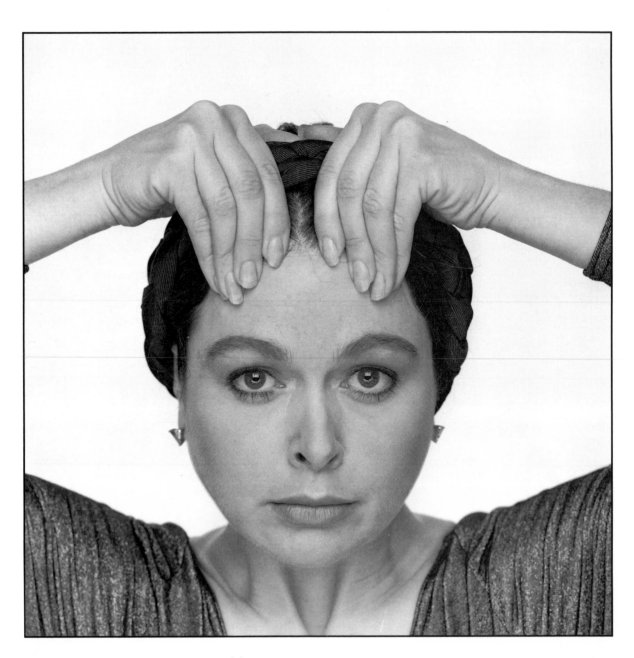

Exercise nineteen
Open the mouth to the shape of 'Ah',
and pull the top mouth and lip
downwards with as much power as
possible, keeping the upper lip tight
against the top teeth. Hold for five-
second contractions, for a duration
of thirty seconds. Put your mind
into it and the exercise then
becomes powerful.

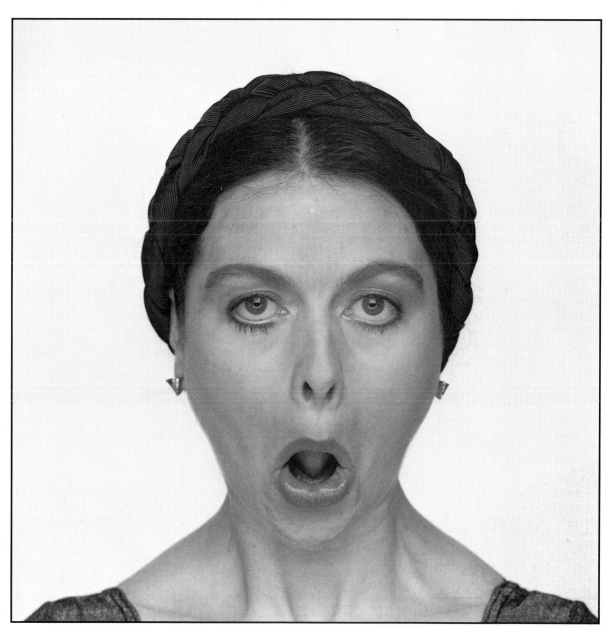

Exercise twenty
Do the exercise quickly: perform thirty 'Ah Hoos' in one exercise period. Open your mouth and mentally say 'Ah', then rapidly, mentally say 'Hoo'. When you say

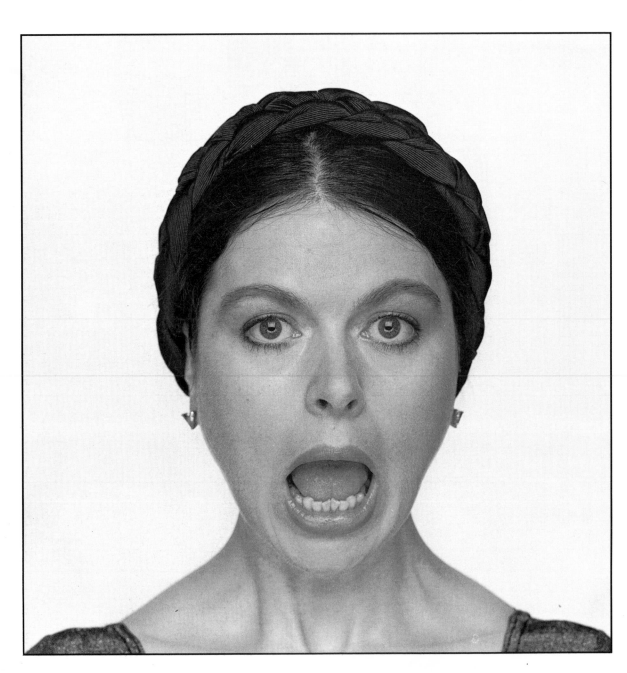

'Ah', open your mouth as wide as possible, and when you say 'Hoo', purse your lips as if you are trying to whistle. Put a lot of power into the exercise.

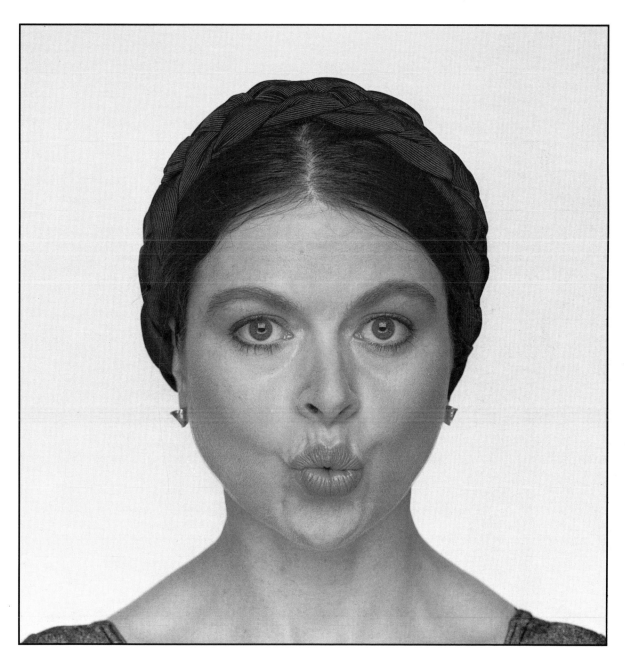

Exercise twenty-one

For this exercise, purse your lips slightly, then pull from the centre of your lips in an outward stretch like an elastic band. Do not part the lips; keep them gently touching each other. Do five-second contractions for thirty seconds.

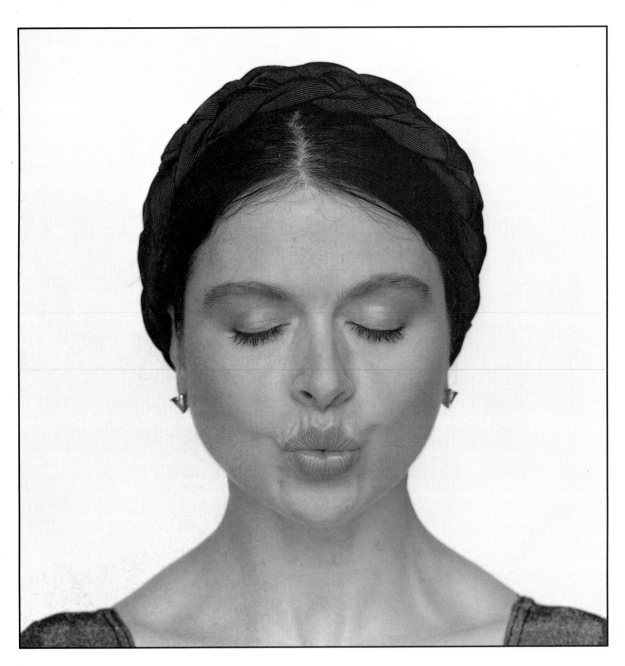

Exercise twenty-two

Place both thumbs into the top lip. Place the first fingers of right and left hands over the top of your thumbs, stretch outwards and down keeping pressure on for five seconds. Slowly relax then perform again. Do this exercise for thirty seconds.

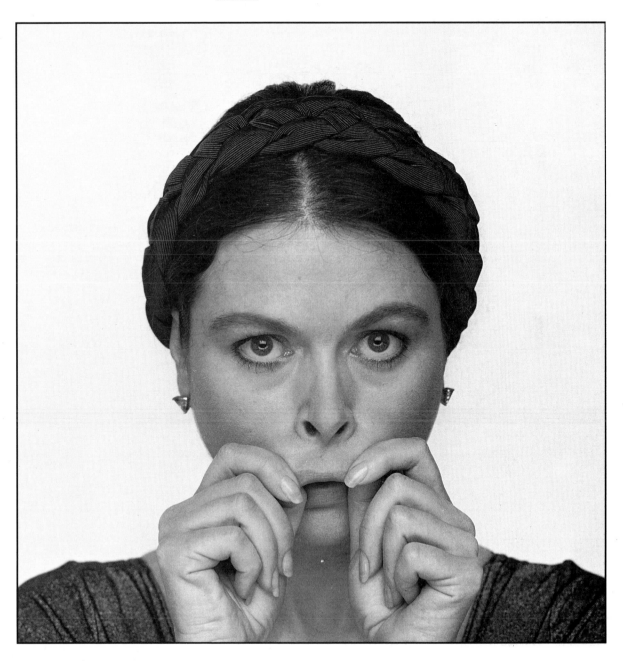

Exercise twenty-three

Put the middle finger of each hand on the beginning of each eyebrow as seen in the photo. Pull eyebrows apart, hold the pressure, and then resist through the muscles in the area with all your will-power. Make it work. Remember that all muscle-building is done through pressure and resistance, and the resistance in muscle-building of the face comes through your mind and will-power. Concentrate on five-second contractions for thirty seconds each day.

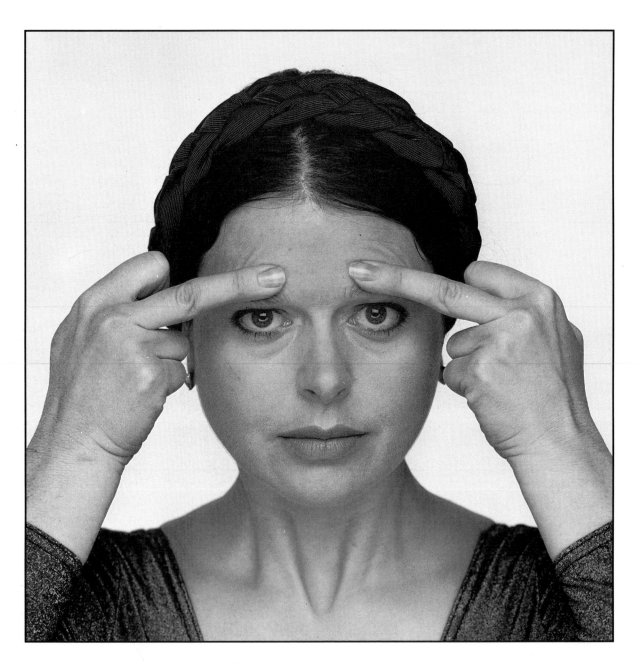

Exercise twenty-four

To have a full, beautiful mouth you need good muscle tone. Bring your teeth together, lips nearly closed, but not tight, slightly relaxed. Now open lips keeping the teeth together, and with your mind and will-power pull the corners of your mouth outwards towards your ears. Concentrate and put some effort into it. Hold the contractions for five-second periods for a total of thirty seconds.

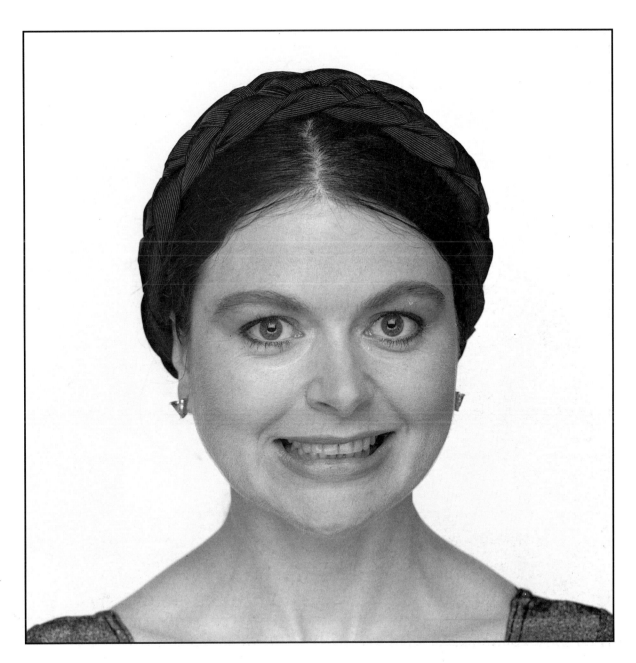

Exercise twenty-five
Open your mouth as wide as
possible in the 'Ah' shape; now
tighten the muscles up and pull out
as hard as you can towards your
ears. Hold for five seconds. Relax
for about five seconds, then repeat
the exercise. Repeat for thirty
seconds.

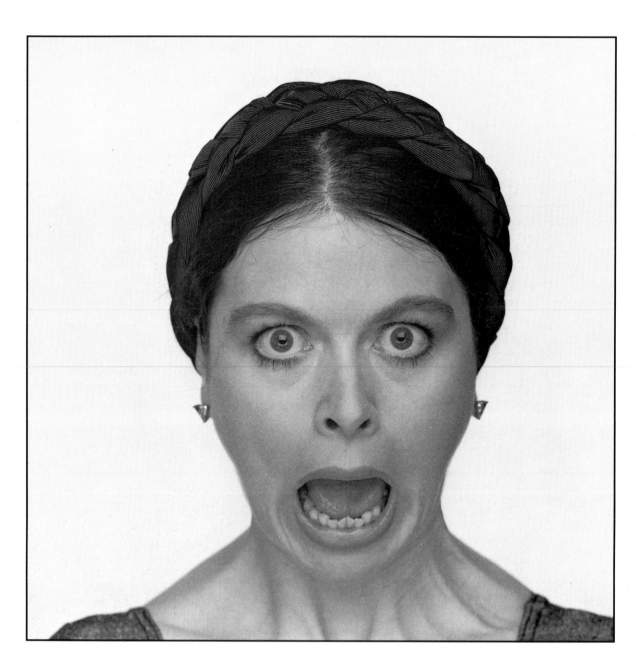

Exercise twenty-six

Place the middle finger of your left hand into the mouth and into the right cheek as seen in the photo. Put pressure on with the finger, your mind completely focused on the area at the same time. Make the muscles of the cheek resist the pressure as you press with your finger. Move your finger on to the different parts of your cheek. Put the pressure on and resist at the same time. Make your mind work. Then place the right hand middle finger into the left cheek and repeat the exercise. Hold the pressure for five-second contractions and repeat for thirty seconds.

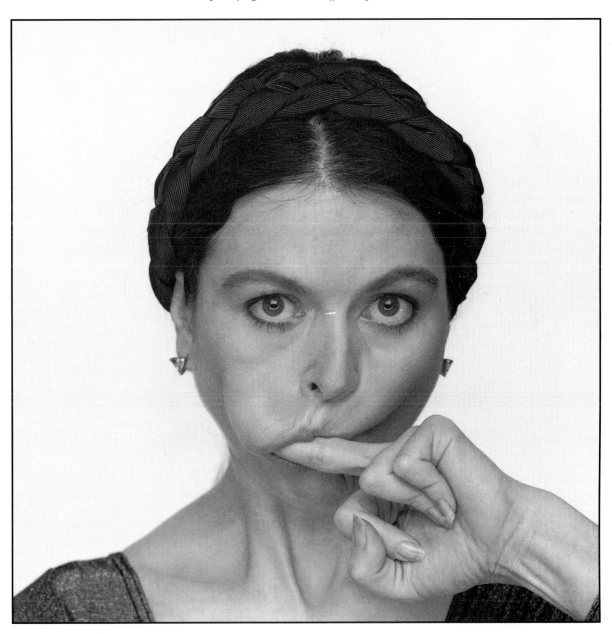

Exercise twenty-seven

Put your thumbs inside your mouth, into the laugh lines on the sides of your face and follow the laugh lines as near to the nose as possible. Then place the first finger of your hands over the thumbs as seen in the photo. Put on the pressure. Now you are putting the pressure on with the thumbs, and you are resisting with the fingers.

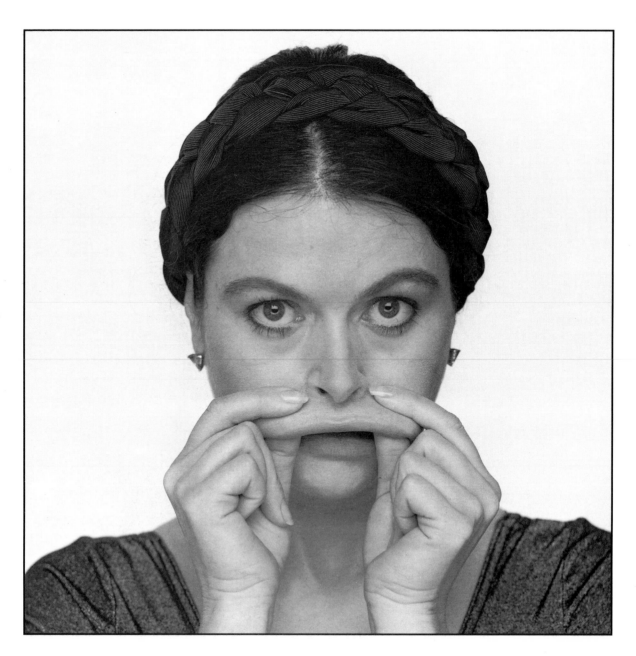

Then release and move your thumbs a little way down the laugh lines and again do a five-second contraction. Do this until you have come all the way down the laugh lines to the corner of the mouth, doing five-second contractions all the way down for thirty seconds.

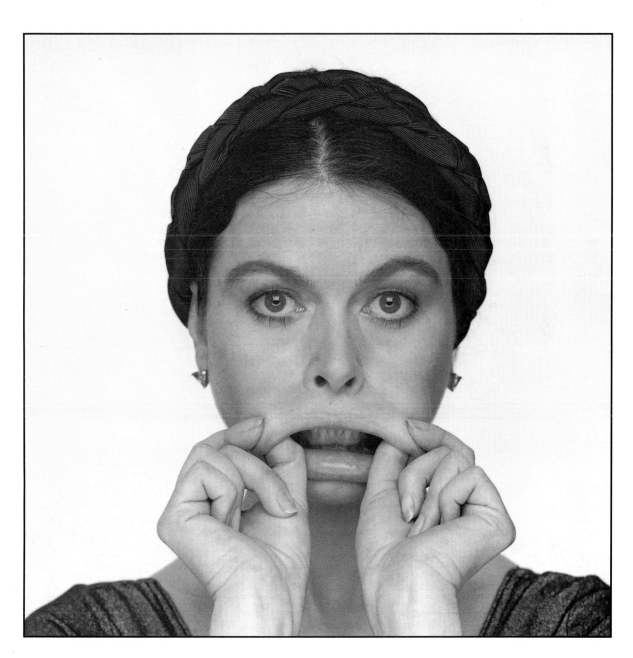

Exercise twenty-eight
Slowly raise the muscles on the right side of your face, from your mouth upwards, until that side of your face is in a big squint. (I find it helpful to sing the scale Do-Re-Me to myself as I tighten the muscles up.)

Hold for five seconds, then

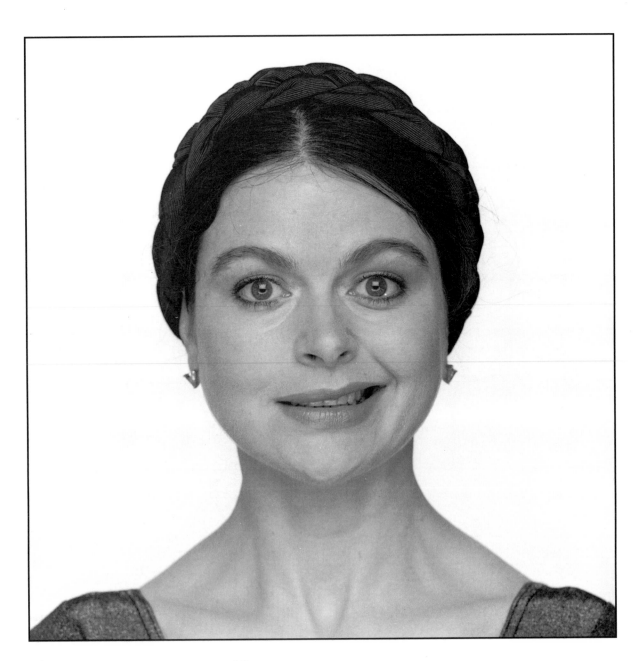

release. Repeat this exercise on the left side of your face. Repeat this exercice six times on each side of your face.

Congratulations! You have just completed Joseph Corvo's twenty-minute Natural Facelift.

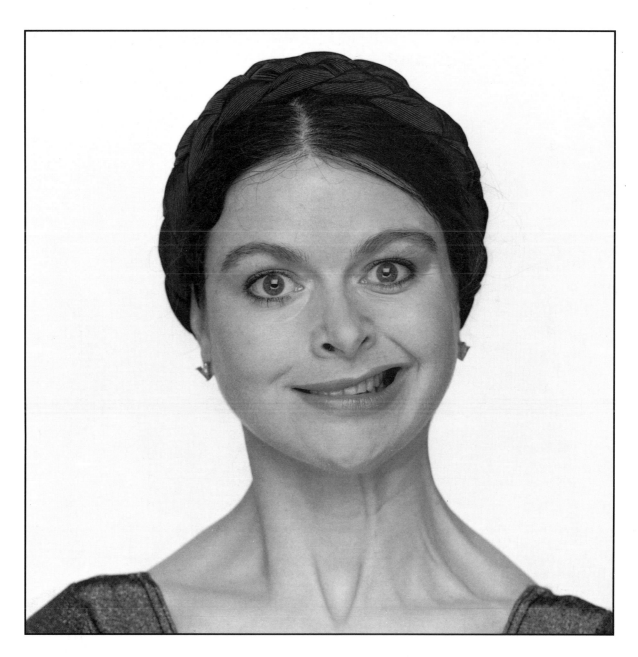

MOISTURIZING

In preparation for your cream, give your face a final toning. Starting from the high mid-point of your forehead and working outwards and downwards, feather your skin with the tips of your fingers. Press up and out, as if flicking the skin off the bone. Work down over your face and then around your neck. But remember that, as with the pressure point massage and the face-building exercises, you must do this as vigorously as possible. This exercise helps to take off the uppermost dead layer of cells.

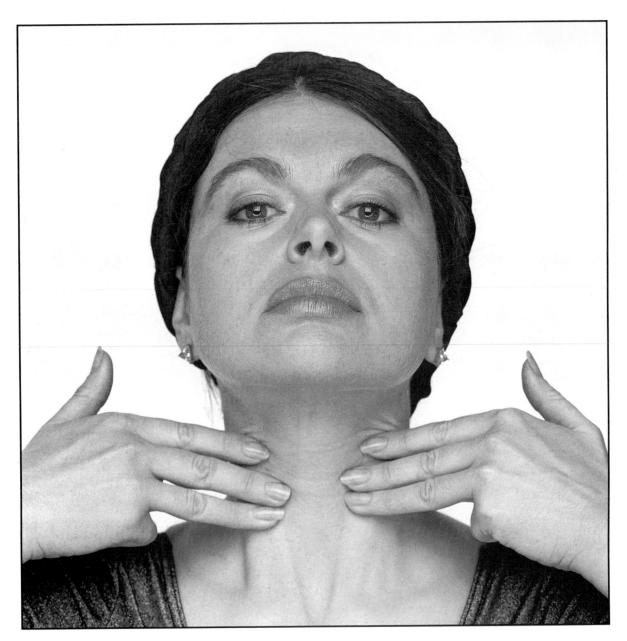

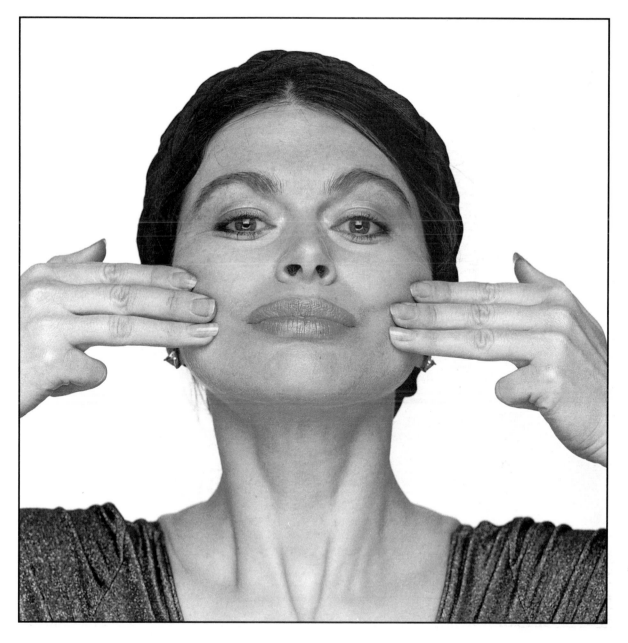

Finally, puff out your cheeks and squeeze your mouth to the size of a pea. Then give your face a good vigorous slapping for two minutes – it will do wonders for your face.

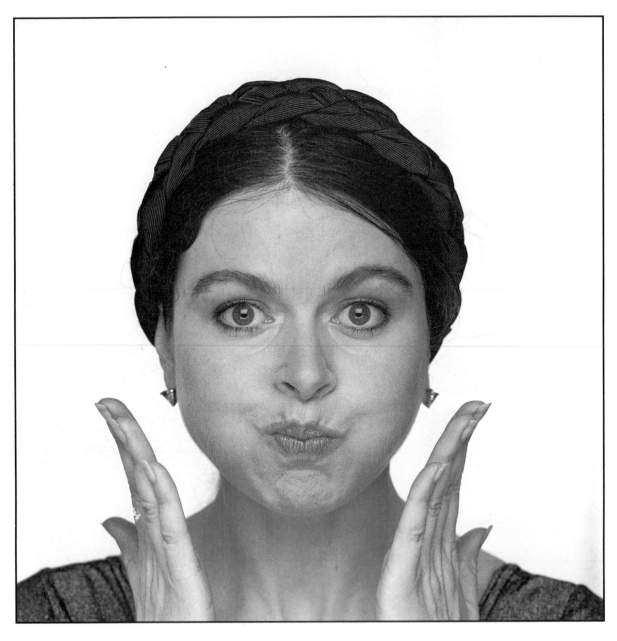

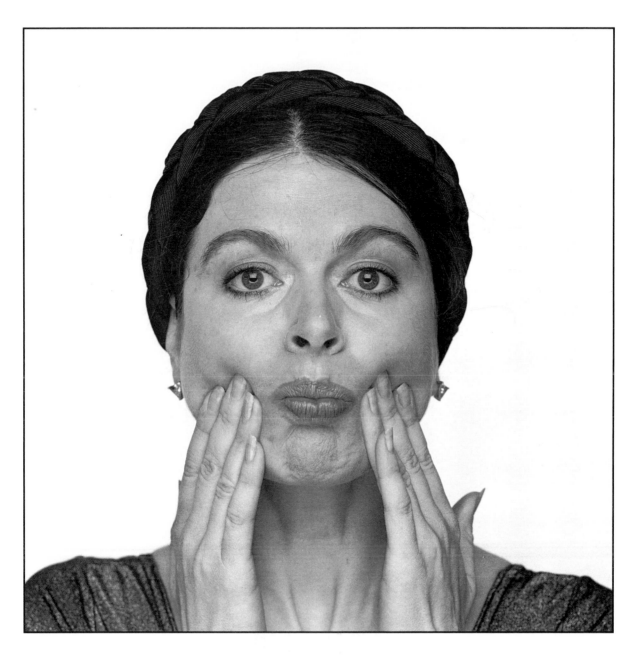

Moisturizing your skin can have a significant role in your beauty treatment. It must be done on a regular basis. If your skin is dry then you should use an oil-based emulsion. Use a light moisturizer if the skin is oily and a richer night cream if you have dry skin. Spread and smooth it on to the face and neck. A good skin and muscle treatment of the face leaves your skin tingling, clean, fresh and absolutely glowing and you look and feel wonderful.

97

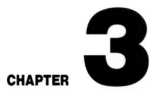

CHAPTER 3

THE ZONE THERAPY LIFESTYLE

**REJUVENATING HABITS
FOR THE REST OF
THE DAY**

There are millions of words of general health advice written every year, and millions of trees destroyed as a result, so I don't want to add to them any more than necessary. But there are certain (commonsensical) things you can refrain from doing in your everyday life so that you don't ruin the work you do in your twenty minutes' exercises.

And there are some positive things you can do which will help your twenty minutes' exercises to keep working for you throughout the day.

DON'T SMOKE
Smoking is very bad for lines on the face. Crows feet deepen. Bags appear under the eyes. The skin becomes grey and lifeless.

DON'T DRINK EXCESSIVELY
The skin becomes pasty and bloated. Veins burst. Too much alcohol causes the liver and kidneys to deteriorate rapidly, and this in turn can ruin the whole glandular and organic system.

DON'T EAT TOO MUCH
Some people have glandular imbalances and malfunctions which Zone Therapy can cure, and Zone Therapy can bring your body to a state of maximum effectiveness in burning off excess weight, but in the main, if you are overweight, there is only one cause – you are eating too much for the amount of exercise you take – and there is only one solution – eat less.

SUNBATHE ONLY IN MODERATION
The sun is particularly dangerous between twelve and three.

NEVER ALLOW WATER TO EVAPORATE ON YOUR SKIN
This causes cracking.

99

MAKE SURE YOU GET AT LEAST EIGHT HOURS' SLEEP

Nine is better. Some people can survive on as few as four hours, but they are burning themselves out and they will suffer in the long run. Lack of sleep makes your face puffy, lifeless, sallow and grey.

UNBLOCK YOUR PORES

Dead cells and dirt tend to block the pores. Blackheads and spots result. Once a week, sit for ten minutes over a bowl of steaming water with a towel covering both your head and the bowl. Afterwards, rinse the face by splashing it with cool water, and then dry it by dabbing it with another, of course dry, towel.

TAKE GOOD CARE OF YOUR TEETH

Always clean your teeth immediately after eating if you can and visit the dentist regularly.

CARE FOR YOUR HAIR

In order to have glorious hair, you must have a healthy scalp, so at least once a week you should massage it either with pure olive oil, slightly warmed, or with almond oil. Next soak a towel in very hot water – not boiling water – then wring the towel out and completely cover the hair with the towel. When the towel cools, repeat the treatment. Then shampoo and dry. Treat your hair gently when you are drying it, because wet hair loses its natural elasticity and can be easily damaged.

This operation should take half an hour. Not only does it ensure a healthy scalp but it relaxes you.

Shining, healthy hair is a reflection of the inner health of your glands and organs and also of good hormone levels. So for glorious hair do your 15 pressure point massage on a daily basis, working particularly on your pituitary gland, your thyroid glands and your adrenal glands.

If you are worried about losing your hair, rub your fingernails together for fifteen minutes each day, simply buffing one set of fingernails against the other.

Foods high in the B vitamins are good for the hair, so eat plenty of liver, kidneys, eggs, wholegrains, yeast extracts, wheat germ and brewer's yeast. Surprising as it may seem, a handful of currants eaten every day is very good for a strong, healthy head of hair.

The way modern life is organized we often find ourselves with useless little bits of time on our hands – odd minutes here and there when it seems impossible to do anything useful. We are caught waiting at the traffic lights, we sit on a tube, we stand in a bus queue. But in fact these odd minutes can be a tremendous opportunity to give ourselves a little tone-up using the pressure points on the hand.

Working with your left hand on your right, move in rotation from the liver to the thyroids to the pituitary gland to the adrenal glands, spending

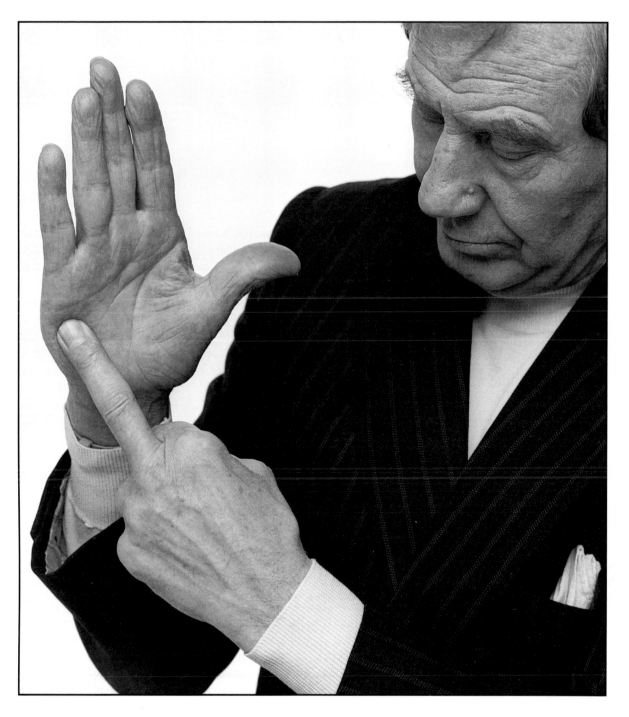

ten seconds on each pressure point before moving on to the next one, and then on until the lights change, the bus arrives or whatever. You will feel a very noticeable effect, even in such a short time.

The Liver will clear your skin.

The Thymus will give you pep.

The Pituitary will give you a relaxed, sexual feeling.

And the Adrenal glands will fill you with energy.

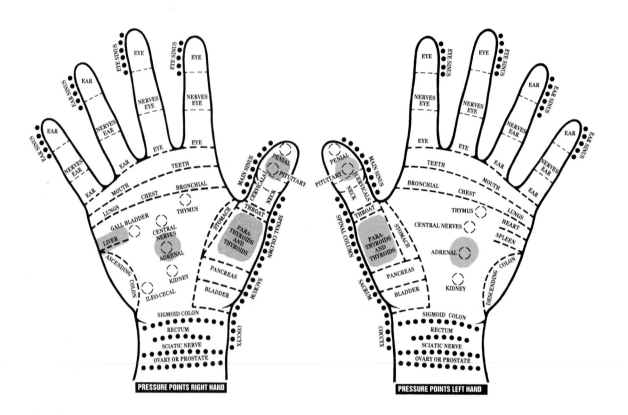

PRESSURE POINTS RIGHT HAND   PRESSURE POINTS LEFT HAND

THE ZONE THERAPY DIET INCLUDING THE LONGEVITY VITAMIN

In order to make the glands and organs work to 100 per cent efficiency, it is very important to feed them properly by eating a balanced diet. You need an abundant supply of proteins, vitamins and minerals.

Proteins, vitamins and minerals are best drawn from natural foods. But if you lead a very busy life, and are sometimes prevented from eating enough of the right kind of food regularly, you will need to supplement your diet. I will tell you how. I will also tell you about the miracle Vitamin B15, and its astonishingly regenerative effect.

PROTEINS

All body tissue is made of protein so it is vital to eat sufficient. When body tissues are not fed sufficient proteins, the normal repair work fails to take place. Muscles become starved so that the body becomes soft and flabby with poor posture.

So to maintain good health and to maximise the effectiveness of your face-building exercises and your pressure point massage, you need up to 95 grammes of protein a day if you are a man and up to 65 grammes a day if you are a woman.

The best sources of protein are chops, kidney, liver and turkey; dairy products such as cheese, cottage cheese, eggs, cream, milk, skimmed-milk, yoghurt; fish proteins such as tuna, salmon, oysters and shrimps; also nuts: peanuts, walnuts, almonds and pecans; vegetables such as beans, soya, dry corn, lentils, potatoes; brewer's yeast, barley bread, whole wheat, oatmeal and rice.

FATS

There is a lot of nonsense talked about cutting fat out of your diet. Fats are the most concentrated form of energy. Fatty acids are needed to help deposit phosphorus in the bones and teeth; they also build resistance to infections and combat tuberculosis. They contain many vital vitamins, particularly in the B group. However, meat fats are much inferior to vegetables in this respect, and they also contribute largely to the formation of cholesterol. So the best fats are soya bean and sunflower oil, wheat germ oil and olive oil.

SUGAR

You also need sugar. Sugars and fat burn together to produce your energy. But do stay clear of refined sugar and take the natural glucose and fructose that can easily be found in most fruit, in dried fruit – apricots, figs and dates are particularly good – and in vegetables such as sweet potatoes and sweet corn and in pure honey and black syrup molasses.

VITAMIN A

Vitamin A is vital for your Natural Facelift. It is terrific in the production of beautiful skin and, before the introduction of fast foods, was largely responsible for what we used to call 'the English Rose complexion'. Vitamin A also helps to give you healthy eyes, and hard nails. A deficiency will cause acne, pale, dry and flaky skin, dry, lifeless hair, dandruff and brittle nails.

You need 10,000–15,000 units a day to complement your Zone Therapy. The best sources are liver, kidney, butter, fish liver oils, carrots, apricots (dried or fresh) and green vegetables. A daily glass of fresh vegetable juice will help you develop the most beautiful complexion.

VITAMIN B

The B vitamins are essential because they have a positive effect on your frame of mind and your moods, giving vitality and energy. Vitamin B2 or riboflavin helps to keep your skin healthy and your eyes bright.

Vitamin B6 keeps the skin beautiful and smooth and also calms the nerves. And Vitamin B is vital in maintaining hair colour.

The best sources are beef, salmon, herring, yeast, brown rice, peas and bananas and black syrup molasses. Wheat germ can be added to cereals and poultry but also to stews. If you are not eating enough of these foods, take a good B-complex pill daily.

VITAMIN C

Vitamin C preserves and enhances your looks, giving elasticity to the body and strength to ligaments, tissues and the walls of blood vessels. It gives you energy and vigour and plays a large part in growth and healing. It protects from illness and fights stress. Without enough of it your skin will age very quickly and develop broken veins. Take at least 200 mg daily.

The best natural sources are, of course, citrus fruits, rosehips, vegetables such as potatoes, broccoli, watercress, parsley, radishes, Brussels sprouts, spinach, tomatoes, turnips and cauliflower. Vitamin C is easily destroyed by cooking, so eat as much in the natural raw state as you can manage. If you think you may not be eating sufficient, it is vital to take a daily supplement in the form of a pill.

VITAMIN D

Vitamin D ensures strong bones and teeth. During the summer months, we will probably get sufficient Vitamin D from the sun. It is also ingested into milk, cream, butter and egg yolk. Other sources of Vitamin D, which may be taken in capsule form, are cod liver oil and halibut liver oil.

VITAMIN E

Vitamin E prolongs the life of the cells in the skin, detoxifying the body in general. It increases sexual and reproductive powers and helps with stress conditions.

The best natural sources are sunflower oil, wheat germ oil, olive oil, oatmeal, yeast, parsley, whole wheat, Brussels sprouts, carrots, asparagus, lettuce, eggs and butter. If you feel you need a supplement, keep below 400 mg in one day.

VITAMIN K

Vitamin K is essential for blood coagulation. The richest sources are cabbage, spinach and carrot tops, all best eaten raw.

CALCIUM AND PHOSPHORUS

Minerals are as important as vitamins for bodily and mental health. Calcium and phosphorus are needed in large quantities to harden the bones and the teeth. Calcium also relaxes the nervous system. The main sources of calcium are milk, buttermilk and yoghurt. Phosphorus is found in dairy products, meat, whole grain and most vegetables. You need at least 800 mg of calcium a day.

IRON

Iron enables the blood to carry oxygen through the body so that energy can be released there. A lack of iron will make you feel tired and listless. The main sources are liver, black syrup molasses, nuts, apricots, wheat bran, wheat germ, carrots, soya beans and peanuts. You need between 10 and 20 milligrams of iron a day if these natural foods are not in your diet regularly.

IODINE

Iodine is essential to vitality. Loss of it causes poor skin, weak muscle tissue and falling hair. The best natural source is seafood, though it is also found in green vegetables and dairy produce.

POTASSIUM

Potassium is essential for energy and clarity of thought. The best sources are whole grain cereals and green vegetables.

THE LONGEVITY VITAMIN

In many parts of the world, including Russia, people regularly take Vitamin B15 for breakfast. Taking regular doses of Vitamin B15 is one of the most effective things you can do to fight against ageing. This miraculous vitamin helps to increase the intake of oxygen into the blood and body tissues, which in turn increases the life span of the cells, and speeds the detoxification of waste. B15 makes the skin tauter and does wonders for the hair. It really does help to make you look years younger.

It originates in the kernel of the apricot stone. The inhabitants of the Hunza region of the Himalayas live to over a hundred years old, and a great many live to one hundred and twenty. Cancer is unknown. One of the main elements of their diet is fresh and dried apricots!

ZONE THERAPY AGAINST COMMON FACIAL PROBLEMS

Particular facial problems are usually caused by the malfunction of a particular gland or organ and by a complementary deficiency in diet. If you suffer from any of the problems described below, your top priority should be to get your whole glandular and organic system working to 100 per cent efficiency again. In addition, pay attention to the items of advice listed below.

ACNE/SPOTS

- boost your intake of Vitamin A
- cleanse your skin on a daily basis by the method described on p. 18
- cleanse your skin on the inside by eating, every day for up to two weeks, five alicante raisins soaked overnight in the juice of a lemon, drinking the lemon juice as well
- massage the following pressure points on your hands

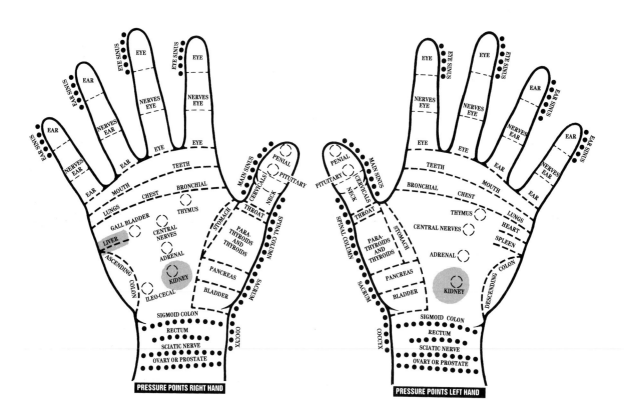

DRY SKIN

- boost your intake of Vitamins E, A, B and C
- cleanse your skin on a daily basis by the method described on p. 18
- during your daily 15 pressure point massage, spend extra time on point 5, which stimulates the sebacious gland, in order to release moisture in the face

BROKEN VEINS

- boost your intake of the B Vitamins
- massage the liver pressure point on your hands and feet

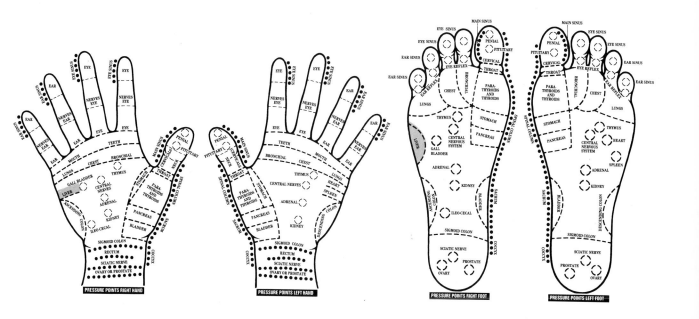

FACIAL HAIR

in women is a result of an imbalance of the gland system as a whole
- in addition to your daily 15 pressure point massage on your face, you should aim to give the pressure points on your feet a thorough workout for five minutes on each foot per day

DULL/TIRED EYES

- boost your intake of Vitamins A and E
- drink eight glasses of water a day
- eat a dish of stewed prunes once a day
- massage the eye pressure points for two minutes on each hand per day
- massage, too, on your right foot, the liver, ascending colon, kidney and sigmoid colon, and on your left foot, your spleen, descending colon and kidney. Work for five minutes on each foot

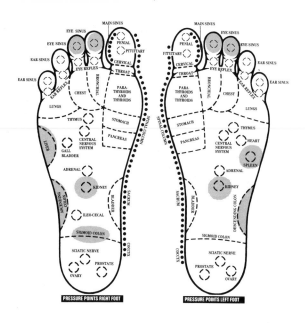

EXCESS FAT

- cut out all chocolate, toffees, sweets, biscuits, cakes, cream, white bread, refined cereals, sugar, potatoes, bread, pasta, rice, bananas, and all alcoholic drink for two months
- maintain meanwhile your intake of protein with cottage cheese, hard-boiled eggs, nuts, soya beans, fish, chicken and lean meats
- maintain high intake of Vitamin C with plenty of fresh fruit and vegetables, particularly red peppers
- take fish liver oil for Vitamin D
- take brewer's yeast for Vitamin B

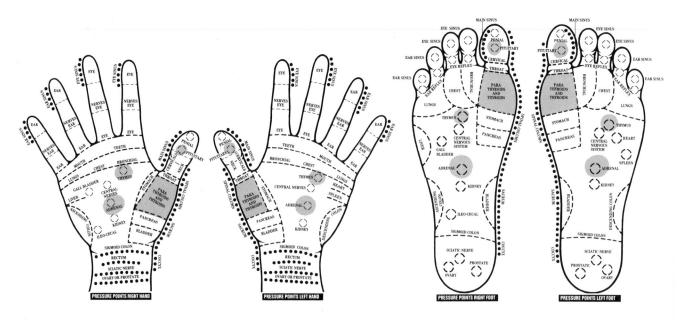

- take 1000 units of Vitamin A per day for ten days
- work the following pressure points for five minutes per day in each hand and foot: thyroid, adrenal glands, thymus and pituitary
- it may be that your lymph glands are not expelling liquid from your body to 100 per cent efficiency, so that you suffer from water retention; cure this by slapping your cheeks as hard as you can for ten minutes a day

ZONE THERAPY'S SEX SECRETS

Being young and being sexy are inextricably linked. I may as well be frank: most of the women who come to me for the Natural Facelift want to look younger so that they can attract men. For them, as for most of us, sexual beauty is the amount of desire that they can generate in the person they desire. We feel marvellous if we inspire that divine vibration in someone!

In fact, to feel beautiful, to *be* beautiful, you must feel sexually desirable, and beyond this to feel sexually fulfilled. Good sex can make you feel wonderful and look beautiful. Sex can be many things – casual, gentle, intense, abandoned, committed, intimate, even fierce – but if it is *good* you will feel happy and relaxed. Good sex makes you sexier.

It is a sad fact, though, that most of the women who come to my clinic, including many of the most beautiful and most famous ones, complain that their partners, though they are kind and gentle, do not satisfy them. The problem is that desire in a man is quicker and more volatile than in a woman. She is calmer and, in a sexual sense, ultimately stronger. Men and women are like fire and water. Fire is quick to ignite but always ultimately overwhelmed by water. Women need longer to become aroused. It is important, then, for the man to exercise control.

So, if you are a man, always be slow and gentle. The slower and gentler you are, the quicker your female partner will become aroused. Do not attempt entry under thirty minutes and then very slowly. If you are becoming over-excited, practise the following exercise.

Breathe in through your nose very slowly – to a count of ten – breathing in to the lower stomach. Do not raise your chest but make sure the breath goes to the stomach. Swallow, then lock your chin into the upper part of your chest and at the same time contract your stomach muscles pushing them outwards. Do not pull your stomach muscles in. Hold for as near as thirty seconds as you can manage.

This exercise will prevent ejaculation.

Get rid of the idea that you must ejaculate because you are making love. In fact it is often more loving *not* to ejaculate. If you have mastered sufficient control to prevent yourself from ejaculating, then you are probably a brilliant, wonderful lover who can always make his partner very happy.

Make love frequently but ejaculate infrequently. In the East they understand that retention of semen is vital to longevity. That is why while we consider a man in his eighties to be extremely old, in China

109

most men live well into their nineties. Your life force of sperm is limited like the sap of a tree. When sap leaves the tree it becomes old and gnarled – and so do men. You only possess so much because as you get older your reproductive system loses its potency. Men over fifty, in particular, should not ejaculate more than once a week, although they may make love every day.

Be careful with your semen and preserve it. Remember what happens to all those old men who marry young girls!

One more Zone Therapy secret. Twelve hundred units of Vitamin E taken one and a half hours before making love ensures a superb sexual performance.

ZONE THERAPY AGAINST STRESS INCLUDING THE ULTIMATE SECRET

Stress is terribly ageing. I have included some anti-stress exercises in the twenty minute daily plan, but if you feel you suffer from stress you will find the following extra exercises extremely helpful. I also include one meditation exercise, though – which I recommend to everyone: I call it the Ultimate Secret.

BREATHING EXERCISES

Exercise one
Lie down on the floor as in the photo. You can put a telephone directory under your head to support your neck if you need it.

Completely relax your toes, feet and ankles, your calves, knees and thighs, your stomach, chest, neck, throat, eyes, ears, hair, shoulders, back, spine, arms, hands and fingers – make this a pleasant sensation.

Take in a breath to a mental count of four. Hold the breath for a mental count of eight. Breathe out to a mental count of four. Try to repeat this exercise five times, aiming eventually to repeat ten times.

After you have mastered the count of four-eight-four, go to six-twelve-six, and eventually on to ten-twenty-ten.

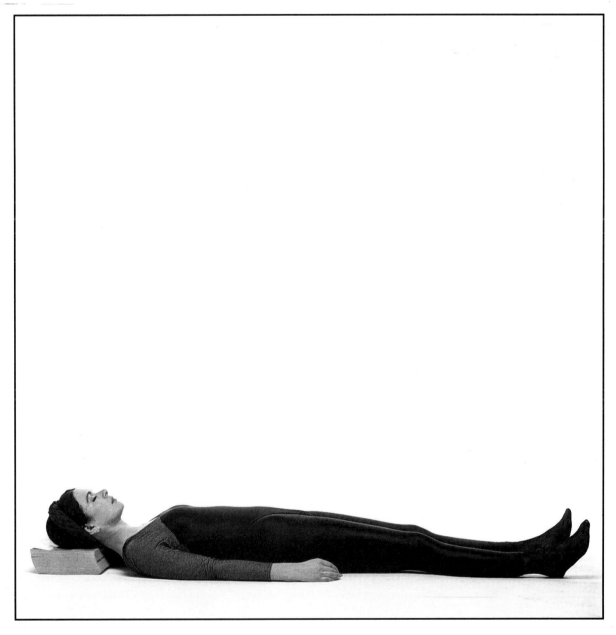

Exercise two

Perform this exercise sitting on the floor in a cross-legged position if possible. If not, sitting properly will do. Place an alarm clock approximately 15 feet away from you. Now concentrate on the ticks, keeping all other thoughts from your mind. You may find it hard to keep all other thoughts from your mind, but apply a little more effort and you will succeed, at least for a few seconds.

Repeat this experiment until you are successful in keeping the mind focused completely and without distraction.

Now let us see what has happened while you have been listening to the ticking sound of the clock. Most of you will have completely suspended the breath; the others who have less concentration must have had very slow breathing.

This proves that where there is concentration of the mind, the breathing becomes very slow or even suspended.

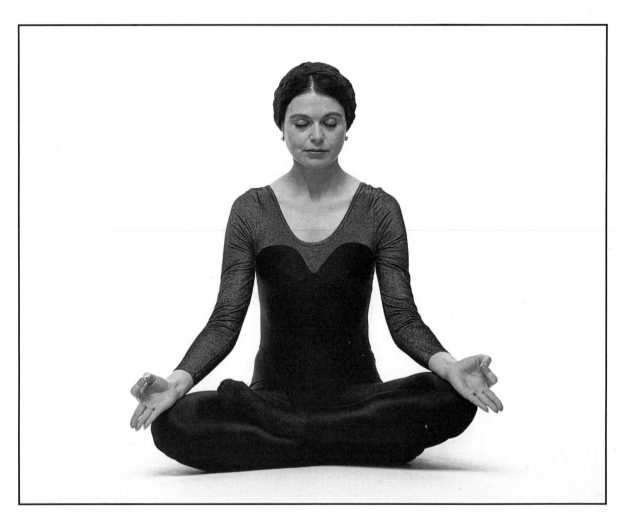

Exercise three

Sit erect, legs crossed if possible – for those unable to sit then take up the corpse pose position as in Exercise 1. Block up the right nostril with the middle finger of the right hand and inhale through the left nostril. Suspend for a mental count of eight and slowly breathe out. Then block up the left nostril with the middle finger of the left hand and inhale slowly. Suspend for a count of eight and slowly breathe out.

Master holding the breath for eight counts, then go on to ten and then twelve until you can master twenty. If you can manage that on a daily basis, I don't think you will be worried by stress.

Exercise four

Sit in a cross-legged position if possible with back straight. Do not use your fingers, use concentration. Inhale through the left nostril, repeating mentally the word 'OM' six times. This will help you enormously with your concentration. Then suspend the breath while you mentally repeat the word 'OM' ten times.

Now exhale through the right nostril while you repeat the word 'OM' six times. Then inhale through the right nostril, repeating 'OM' six times. Suspend the breath mentally counting 'OM' ten times. Exhale counting 'OM' six times and repeat.

You really must concentrate to make certain you are isolating one nostril whilst breathing in and also breathing out.

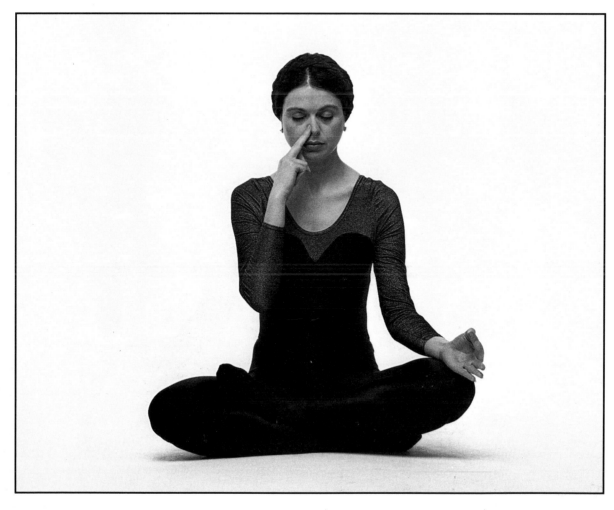

Exercise five

In a sitting position close the right nostril with your right thumb and inhale through the left nostril. Now close the left nostril immediately with your right ring finger. Remove your thumb from the right nostril and exhale through that nostril. This is half a round.

Now, without pausing, inhale through the right nostril, close the right nostril with your right thumb and inhale through the left nostril. This makes one full round. Repeat for six rounds if possible.

Concentration and a sense of peace are what you will develop over a period of time, peace and tranquillity.

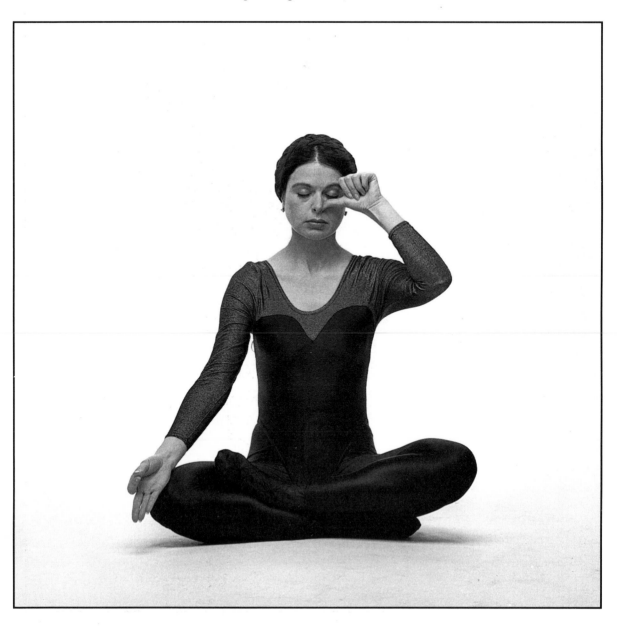

Position 1

The Sun Exercise
If done in the morning, face the sun.
Stand as in the photo. Put the
hands together as in prayer,
standing with the feet together.

THE PRACTICE OF RELAXATION
We need physical exercise to help the body relax and to remove tension.

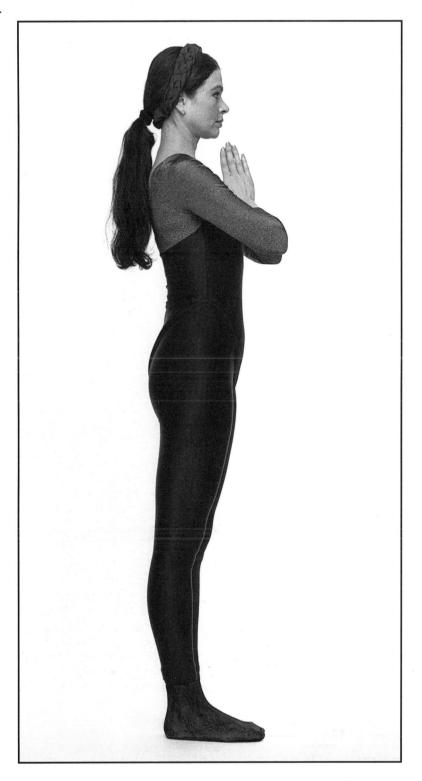

Position 2
*Inhale and raise the arms and bend
backwards as in the photo.*

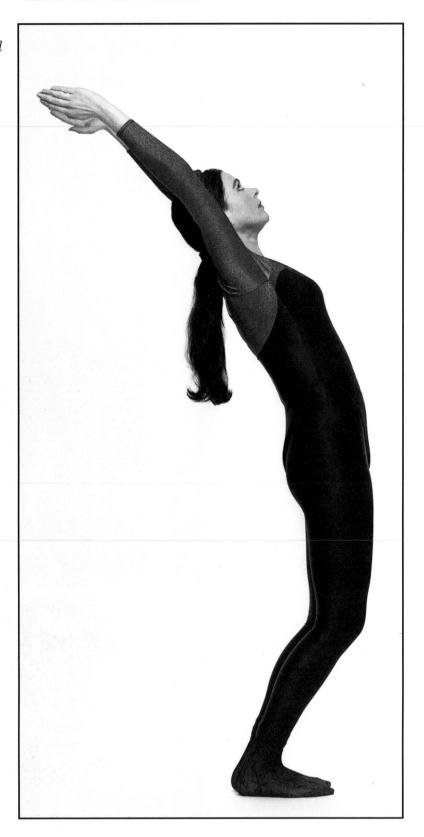

Position 3

Exhale and bend forward till the hands are in line with the feet. Try to touch the knees with your head. In the beginning the knees may be slightly bent until the head can touch them. After some practice the knees should be straightened.

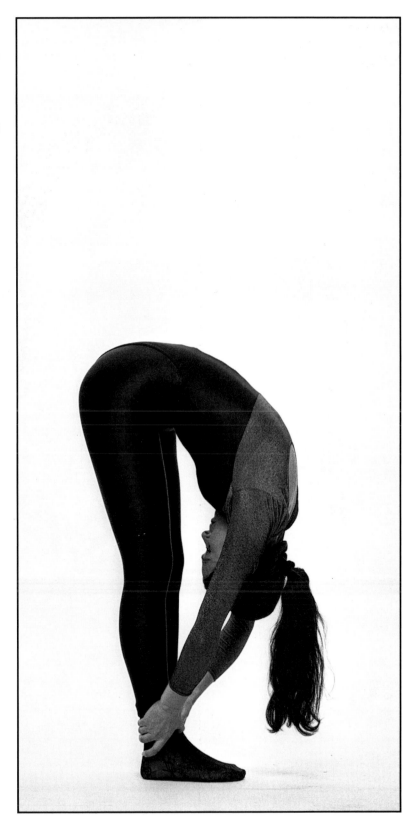

Position 4
*Inhale and move the right leg away
from the body in a big backward
step. Keep the hands and left foot
firmly on the ground. Bending the
head backward, the left knee should
be between the arms.*

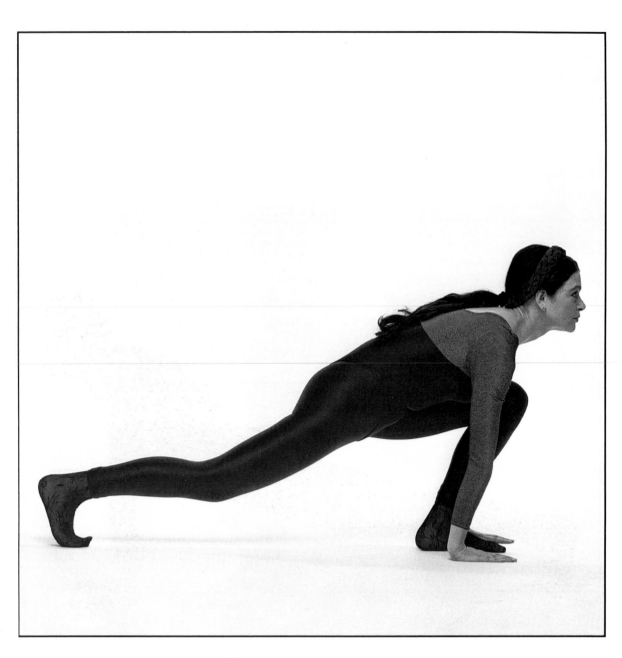

Position 5
*Inhale and hold the breath. Move
the left leg from the body and
keeping both feet together and the
knees off the floor, rest on the hands
(arms straight) and keep the body
in a straight line from head to foot.*

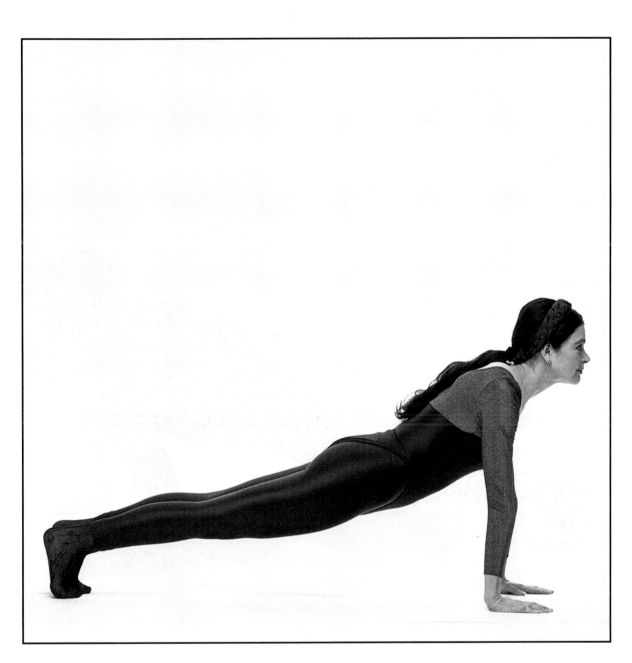

Position 6
*Exhale and lower the body to the
floor. In this position, known as the
eight-curved prostration, only eight
portions of the body come in contact
with the floor; two feet, two knees,
two hands, chest and forehead. The
abdominal region is raised and, if
possible, the nose is also kept off the
floor, the forehead only touching it.*

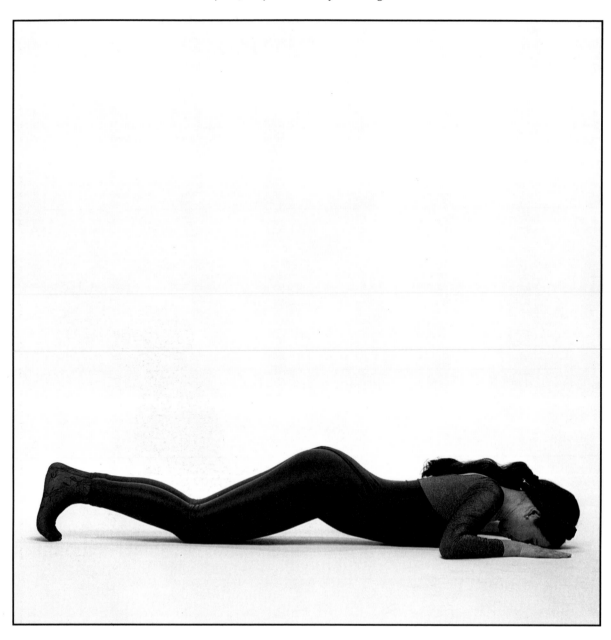

Position 7
Inhale and bend backward as much as possible, bending the spine to the maximum.

Position 8
Exhale and lift the body. Keep the feet and heels flat on the floor.

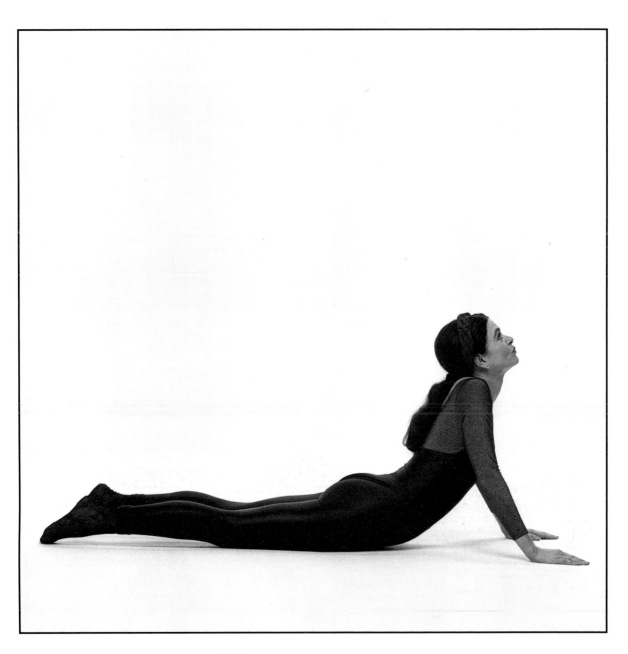

Position 9
Inhale and bring the right foot
along the level of the hands. The
left foot and knee should touch the
ground, looking up bending the
spine slightly.

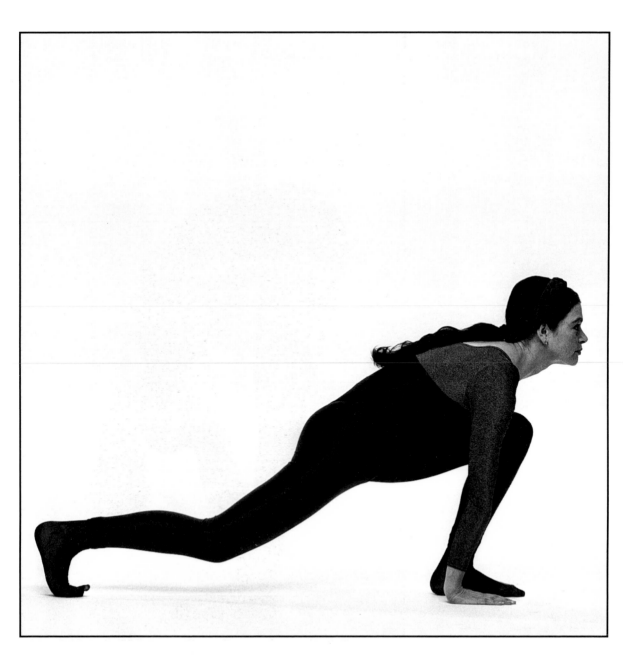

Position 10
Exhale and bring the left leg forward, keeping the knees straight and bringing the head down to the knees as in the third position.

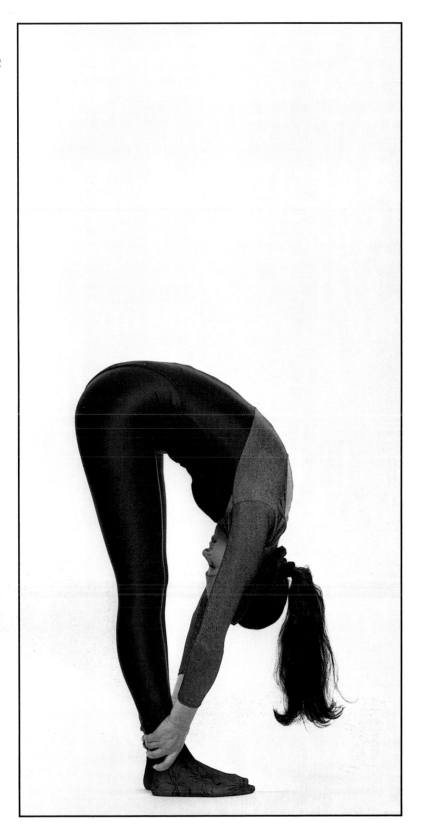

Position 11
Raise the arms overhead and bend backward inhaling as in Position 2.

Position 12
Exhale. Drop the arms and relax. Repeat these exercises as many times as you feel like.

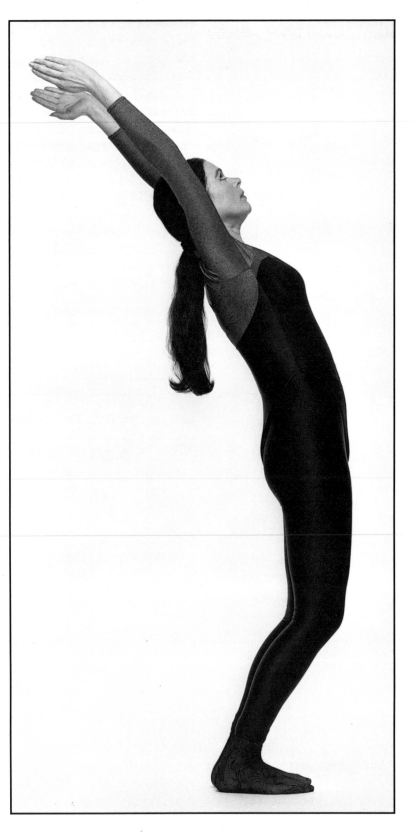

The ladder from which one falls, so to speak, is the same ladder that leads one up. The imagination that is needed for the liberation of the soul is just the same imagination that produces base, worldly thoughts, enslaves, binds, and keeps one at the mercy of all circumstances.

A man dreams, and in his dreams all sorts of things appear. The things in the dream are mere ideas, mere thoughts and imagination. Yet for the person dreaming, a tiger or a lion in a dream can be as real as a living one, and he is startled and awakened. But as soon as he is awake, fear of the tiger or lion vanishes and without further explanation he knows that all the objects in the dream world were unreal.

Similarly, the whole world is a dream. The pictures of birth and death, big and small, rich and poor, good and evil, pain and pleasure, are nothing but false imagination.

The practice of pure godliness leads one to that place where all imagination ceases, where all language ceases, in which there remains only that one indescribable reality. In that state there is no more birth or death for the soul, and the soul shines in itself.

MEDITATION

This meditation should be started after a few rounds of breathing exercises.

The aim is to make the mind rise into the higher regions. This can be done by humming the syllable 'OM'.

The meaning of the syllable 'OM' is different to different persons. Everyone in his own stage of spiritual development has to give it the meaning that suits him or her best. Some people meditate on 'OM' as the Sun of Suns shining within their hearts. While others meditate on the space between the eyebrows. But I recommend that when you start practising this exercise, you should think on the following meditation as you chant 'OM':

> I am the light of lights. I am the real sun. It is I who appear in all the beautiful flowers. In me the whole world lives, moves, and has its being. I am manifested everywhere. I existed before the world began.

> Evil thoughts and worldly desires are things concerning the false body and the false mind and are things of darkness.

> I command elements. I am all-pervading like light and invisible rays. I permeate every atom and every object.

> I am the lowest. I am the highest. I am the showman. I am the spectator. I am the performer.

> I am the most famous people and the most disreputable and ignominious. I am the most fallen. I am the most beautiful. I shine in the lightning. I roar in the thunder. I flutter in the leaves. I whisper in the winds. I roll in the surging seas. I am friend. I am foe. I am ALL.

> I am the whole universe. Everything is in me. I am limitless, eternal, all-pervading, I am in you, you are in me.

CHAPTER **4**

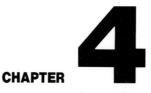

FINAL MESSAGE FROM JOSEPH CORVO

Take responsibility for your health now. It is your highest duty, because unless you are in the best condition it is possible for you to be, you will be unable to do anything else 100 per cent.

We all tend to fool ourselves when we look in the mirror, so I suggest you take a photograph of yourself now, then another one after three months of practising the exercises in this book. What you will see will not be mere cosmetic beauty, but the beauty that comes from deep health and the positive attitude that springs from it.

Zone Therapy is miraculous. The results will astonish you.

Once more, dear friends, I end this book in the greatest hope that within its contents there is something for all of you. Something that will bring you great beauty of face, body, mind and spirit – whatever it is you are searching for – and with God's blessing may you find it.

Joseph Corvo